SpringerBriefs in Applied Sciences and Technology

Computational Intelligence

Series Editor

Janusz Kacprzyk, Systems Research Institute, Polish Academy of Sciences, Warsaw, Poland

SpringerBriefs in Computational Intelligence are a series of slim high-quality publications encompassing the entire spectrum of Computational Intelligence. Featuring compact volumes of 50 to 125 pages (approximately 20,000-45,000 words), Briefs are shorter than a conventional book but longer than a journal article. Thus Briefs serve as timely, concise tools for students, researchers, and professionals.

More information about this subseries at http://www.springer.com/series/10618

Simon James Fong · Nilanjan Dey ·
Jyotismita Chaki

Artificial Intelligence
for Coronavirus Outbreak

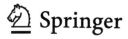 Springer

Simon James Fong
Department of Computer
and Information Science
University of Macau
Taipa, Macau, China

Nilanjan Dey
Department of Information Technology
Techno International New Town
Kolkata, West Bengal, India

Jyotismita Chaki
School of Information Technology
and Engineering
Vellore Institute of Technology
Vellore, Tamil Nadu, India

ISSN 2191-530X   ISSN 2191-5318   (electronic)
SpringerBriefs in Applied Sciences and Technology
ISSN 2625-3704   ISSN 2625-3712   (electronic)
SpringerBriefs in Computational Intelligence
ISBN 978-981-15-5935-8   ISBN 978-981-15-5936-5   (eBook)
https://doi.org/10.1007/978-981-15-5936-5

This Springer imprint is published by the registered company Springer Nature Singapore Pte Ltd.
The registered company address is: 152 Beach Road, #21-01/04 Gateway East, Singapore 189721, Singapore

Preface

This book shows a buffet of artificial intelligence applications from drones to deep learning and from data analysis to the prediction of the next pandemic disease along with its drug discovery. Today the entire globe is under the threat of COVID-19 affecting around 200 countries. The death toll reported in these highly affected countries has become catastrophic. Countries next in line where the pandemic is still in the second stage are closely monitored to check and create a barrier where there lies a severe chance of community spread. Here, close monitoring of sensitive regions using drones and modelling of the prediction mechanism to visualize the extent and severity of the spread of the disease within the community are highly required. Effective usage of drones has been reported encompassing community monitoring during lockdown to sanitization of the highly susceptible and the next probable hotspots. On the other hand, data analysis plays a pivotal role to understand the nature and the potential ability of community spreading. Although several drugs that are administered to treat some major diseases in the developing nations are currently undergoing clinical trials and various tests for their curative efficacy towards the disease, and several promising results have come to the fore, nailing down to the vaccine is still an uphill task. Anticipating a future where AI applications will evolve and enhance to serve mankind.

Chapter 1 provides an introduction to the coronavirus outbreak (COVID-19). A brief history of this virus along with the symptoms are reported in this chapter. Then the comparison between COVID-19 and other plagues is included in this chapter. Reviews of online portals and social media are reported in this chapter. Also, the preventive measures and policies enforced by the WHO and different countries are included in this chapter. Emergency funding provided by different countries to fight the COVID-19 is mentioned in this chapter. Lastly, artificial intelligence, data science, and technological solutions are included in this chapter.

Chapter 2 includes infection risk identification and smart screening for high body temperature. Also, deep learning, AI-driven unmanned technologies, and radiological image analysis related to COVID-19 are discussed in this chapter.

AI-empowered data analytics for coronavirus epidemic monitoring and control are discussed in chapter 3. This chapter introduces and discusses how some of the prominent AI and data analytics examples crunch over the data during COVID-19, for forecast and insights.

Finally, Chap. 4 concludes the book and summarizes the book content.

Taipa, Macau, China   Simon James Fong
Kolkata, India   Nilanjan Dey
Vellore, India   Jyotismita Chaki

Contents

About the Authors

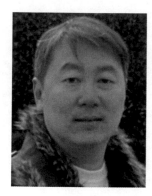

Dr. Simon James Fong graduated from La Trobe University, Australia, with a 1st Class Honours BEng. Computer Systems degree and a PhD. Computer Science degree in 1993 and 1998 respectively. Simon is now working as an Associate Professor at the Computer and Information Science Department of the University of Macau, as an Adjunct Professor at Faculty of Informatics, Durban University of Technology, South Africa, at ZIAT of Chinese Academy of Science, and at Department of Computer Science, Xi'an Polytechnic University, Xi'an, China. He is a co-founder of the Data Analytics and Collaborative Computing Research Group in the Faculty of Science and Technology. Prior to his academic career, Simon took up various managerial and technical posts, such as systems engineer, IT consultant and e-commerce director in Australia and Asia. Dr. Fong has published over 450 international conference and peer-reviewed journal papers, mostly in the areas of data mining, data stream mining, big data analytics, meta-heuristics optimization algorithms, and their applications. He serves on the editorial boards of the Journal of Network and Computer Applications of Elsevier, IEEE IT Professional Magazine, and various special issues of SCIE-indexed journals. Simon is also an active researcher with leading positions such as Vice-chair of IEEE Computational Intelligence Society (CIS) Task Force on "Business Intelligence & Knowledge Management", TC Chair of

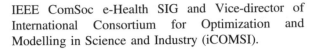

IEEE ComSoc e-Health SIG and Vice-director of International Consortium for Optimization and Modelling in Science and Industry (iCOMSI).

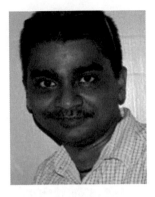

Dr. Nilanjan Dey is an Assistant Professor in the Department of Information Technology at Techno International New Town (Formerly known as Techno India College of Technology), Kolkata, India. He is a visiting fellow of the University of Reading, UK. He was an honorary Visiting Scientist at Global Biomedical Technologies Inc., CA, USA (2012–2015). He was awarded his PhD from Jadavpur University in 2015. He is the Editor-in-Chief of the International Journal of Ambient Computing and Intelligence, IGI Global. He is the Series Co-Editor of Springer Tracts in Nature-Inspired Computing, Springer Nature, Series Co-Editor of Advances in Ubiquitous Sensing Applications for Healthcare, Elsevier, Series Editor of Computational Intelligence in Engineering Problem Solving and Intelligent Signal processing and data analysis, CRC. He has authored/edited more than 75 books with Springer, Elsevier, Wiley, CRC Press, and published more than 300 peer-reviewed research papers. His main research interests include Medical Imaging, Machine learning, Computer-Aided Diagnosis, Data Mining, etc. He is the Indian Ambassador of the International Federation for Information Processing (IFIP) – Young ICT Group.

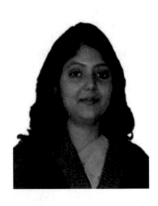

Dr. Jyotismita Chaki is an Assistant Professor in School of Information Technology and Engineering at Vellore Institute of Technology, Vellore, India. She has done her PhD (Engg) from Jadavpur University, Kolkata, India. Her research interests include: Computer Vision and Image Processing, Artificial Intelligence, Pattern Recognition, Medical Imaging, Soft computing, Data mining, Machine learning. She has authored many international conferences and journal papers. She is the author of the following books titled: (1) A Beginner's Guide to Image Preprocessing Techniques (CRC Press, Taylor and Francis), (2) A Beginner's Guide to Image Shape Feature Extraction Techniques (CRC Press, Taylor and Francis) and (3) Texture Feature Extraction Techniques for Image

Recognition (Springer). She has served as a reviewer of Applied Soft Computing (Elsevier), Biosystem Engineering (Elsevier), Pattern Recognition Letters (Elsevier), Journal of Visual Communication and Image Representation (Elsevier), Signal Image and Video Processing (Springer) journal and also served as Program Committee member of many reputed conferences.

Chapter 1
An Introduction to COVID-19

1.1 A Brief History of the Coronavirus Outbreak

A novel coronavirus (CoV) named '2019-nCoV' or '2019 novel coronavirus' or 'COVID-19' by the World Health Organization (WHO) is in charge of the current outbreak of pneumonia that began at the beginning of December 2019 near in Wuhan City, Hubei Province, China [1–4]. COVID-19 is a pathogenic virus. From the phylogenetic analysis carried out with obtainable full genome sequences, bats occur to be the COVID-19 virus reservoir, but the intermediate host(s) has not been detected till now. Though three major areas of work already are ongoing in China to advise our awareness of the pathogenic origin of the outbreak. These include early inquiries of cases with symptoms occurring near in Wuhan during December 2019, ecological sampling from the Huanan Wholesale Seafood Market as well as other area markets, and the collection of detailed reports of the point of origin and type of wildlife species marketed on the Huanan market and the destination of those animals after the market has been closed [5–8].

Coronaviruses mostly cause gastrointestinal and respiratory tract infections and are inherently categorized into four major types: Gammacoronavirus, Deltacoronavirus, Betacoronavirus and Alphacoronavirus [9–11]. The first two types mainly infect birds, while the last two mostly infect mammals. Six types of human CoVs have been formally recognized. These comprise HCoVHKU1, HCoV-OC43, Middle East Respiratory Syndrome coronavirus (MERS-CoV), Severe Acute Respiratory Syndrome coronavirus (SARS-CoV) which is the type of the Betacoronavirus, HCoV229E and HCoV-NL63, which are the member of the Alphacoronavirus. Coronaviruses did not draw global concern until the 2003 SARS pandemic [12–14], preceded by the 2012 MERS [15–17] and most recently by the COVID-19 outbreaks. SARS-CoV and MERS-CoV are known to be extremely pathogenic and spread from bats to palm civets or dromedary camels and eventually to humans.

COVID-19 is spread by dust particles and fomites while close unsafe touch between the infector and the infected individual. Airborne distribution has not been recorded for COVID-19 and is not known to be a significant transmission engine based on empirical evidence; although it can be imagined if such aerosol-generating practices are carried out in medical facilities. Faecal spreading has been seen in certain patients, and the active virus has been reported in a small number of clinical studies [18–20]. Furthermore, the faecal-oral route does not seem to be a COVID-19 transmission engine; its function and relevance for COVID-19 need to be identified.

For about 18,738,58 laboratory-confirmed cases recorded as of 2nd week of April 2020, the maximum number of cases (77.8%) was between 30 and 69 years of age. Among the recorded cases, 21.6% are farmers or employees by profession, 51.1% are male and 77.0% are Hubei.

However, there are already many concerns regarding the latest coronavirus. Although it seems to be transferred to humans by animals, it is important to recognize individual animals and other sources, the path of transmission, the incubation cycle, and the features of the susceptible community and the survival rate. Nonetheless, very little clinical knowledge on COVID-19 disease is currently accessible and details on age span, the animal origin of the virus, incubation time, outbreak curve, viral spectroscopy, dissemination pathogenesis, autopsy observations, and any clinical responses to antivirals are lacking among the serious cases.

1.2 How Different and Deadly COVID-19 is Compared to Plagues in History

COVID-19 has reached to more than 150 nations, including China, and has caused WHO to call the disease a worldwide pandemic. By the time of 2nd week of April 2020, this COVID-19 cases exceeded 18,738,58, although more than 1,160,45 deaths were recorded worldwide and United States of America became the global epicentre of coronavirus. More than one-third of the COVID-19 instances are outside of China. Past pandemics that have existed in the past decade or so, like bird flu, swine flu, and SARS, it is hard to find out the comparison between those pandemics and this coronavirus. Following is a guide to compare coronavirus with such diseases and recent pandemics that have reformed the world community.

1.2.1 Coronavirus Versus Seasonal Influenza

Influenza, or seasonal flu, occurs globally every year–usually between December and February. It is impossible to determine the number of reports per year because it is not a reportable infection (so no need to be recorded to municipality), so often patients with minor symptoms do not go to a physician. Recent figures placed the Rate of Case Fatality at 0.1% [21–23].

There are approximately 3–5 million reports of serious influenza a year, and about 250,000–500,000 deaths globally. In most developed nations, the majority of deaths arise in persons over 65 years of age. Moreover, it is unsafe for pregnant mothers, children under 59 months of age and individuals with serious illnesses.

The annual vaccination eliminates infection and severe risks in most developing countries but is nevertheless a recognized yet uncomfortable aspect of the season.

In contrast to the seasonal influenza, coronavirus is not so common, has led to fewer cases till now, has a higher rate of case fatality and has no antidote.

1.2.2   Coronavirus Versus Bird Flu (H5N1 and H7N9)

Several cases of bird flu have existed over the years, with the most severe in 2013 and 2016. This is usually from two separate strains—H5N1 and H7N9 [24–26].

The H7N9 outbreak in 2016 accounted for one-third of all confirmed human cases but remained confined relative to both coronavirus and other pandemics/outbreak cases. After the first outbreak, about 1,233 laboratory-confirmed reports of bird flu have occurred. The disease has a Rate of Case Fatality of 20–40%.

Although the percentage is very high, the blowout from individual to individual is restricted, which, in effect, has minimized the number of related deaths. It is also impossible to monitor as birds do not necessarily expire from sickness.

In contrast to the bird flu, coronavirus becomes more common, travels more quickly through human to human interaction, has an inferior cardiothoracic ratio, resulting in further total fatalities and spread from the initial source.

1.2.3   Coronavirus Versus Ebola Epidemic

The Ebola epidemic of 2013 was primarily centred in 10 nations, including Sierra Leone, Guinea and Liberia have the greatest effects, but the extremely high Case Fatality Rate of 40% has created this as a significant problem for health professionals nationwide [27–29].

Around 2013 and 2016, there were about 28,646 suspicious incidents and about 11,323 fatalities, although these are expected to be overlooked. Those who survived from the original epidemic may still become sick months or even years later, because the infection may stay inactive for prolonged periods. Thankfully, a vaccination was launched in December 2016 and is perceived to be effective.

In contrast to the Ebola, coronavirus is more common globally, has caused in fewer fatalities, has a lesser case fatality rate, has no reported problems during treatment and after recovery, does not have an appropriate vaccination.

1.2.4   Coronavirus Versus Camel Flu (MERS)

Camel flu is a misnomer–though camels have MERS antibodies and may have been included in the transmission of the disease; it was originally transmitted to humans through bats [30–32]. Like Ebola, it infected only a limited number of nations, i.e. about 27, but about 858 fatalities from about 2,494 laboratory-confirmed reports suggested that it was a significant threat if no steps were taken in place to control it.

In contrast to the camel flu, coronavirus is more common globally, has occurred more fatalities, has a lesser case fatality rate, and spreads more easily among humans.

1.2.5   Coronavirus Versus Swine Flu (H1N1)

Swine flu is the same form of influenza that wiped 1.7% of the world population in 1918. This was deemed a pandemic again in June 2009 an approximately-21% of the global population infected by this [33–35].

Thankfully, the case fatality rate is substantially lower than in the last pandemic, with 0.1%–0.5% of events ending in death. About 18,500 of these fatalities have been laboratory-confirmed, but statistics range as high as 151,700–575,400 world-wide. 50–80% of severe occurrences have been reported in individuals with chronic illnesses like asthma, obesity, cardiovascular diseases and diabetes.

In contrast to the swine flu, coronavirus is not so common, has caused fewer fatalities, has more case fatality rate, has a longer growth time and less impact on young people.

1.2.6   Coronavirus Versus Severe Acute Respiratory Syndrome (SARS)

SARS was discovered in 2003 as it spread from bats to humans resulted in about 774 fatalities. By May there were eventually about 8,100 reports across 17 countries, with a 15% case fatality rate. The number is estimated to be closer to 9.6% as confirmed cases are counted, with 0.9% cardiothoracic ratio for people aged 20–29, rising to 28% for people aged 70–79. Similar to coronavirus, SARS had bad results for males than females in all age categories [36–38].

Coronavirus is more common relative to SARS, which ended in more overall fatalities, lower case fatality rate, the even higher case fatality rate in older ages, and poorer results for males.

1.2.7 Coronavirus Versus Hong Kong Flu (H3N2)

The Hong Kong flu pandemic erupted on 13 July 1968, with 1–4 million deaths globally by 1969. It was one of the greatest flu pandemics of the twentieth century, but thankfully the case fatality rate was smaller than the epidemic of 1918, resulting in fewer fatalities overall. That may have been attributed to the fact that citizens had generated immunity owing to a previous epidemic in 1957 and to better medical treatment [39].

In contrast to the Hong Kong flu, coronavirus is not so common, has caused in fewer fatalities and has a higher case fatality rate.

1.2.8 Coronavirus Versus Spanish Flu (H1N1)

The 1918 Spanish flu pandemic was one of the greatest occurrences of recorded history. During the first year of the pandemic, lifespan in the US dropped by 12 years, with more civilians killed than HIV/AIDS in 24 h [40–42].

Regardless of the name, the epidemic did not necessarily arise in Spain; wartime censors in Germany, the United States, the United Kingdom and France blocked news of the disease, but Spain did not, creating the misleading perception that more cases and fatalities had occurred relative to its neighbours

This strain of H1N1 eventually affected more than 500 million men, or 27% of the world's population at the moment, and had deaths of between 40 and 50 million. At the end of 1920, 1.7% of the world's people had expired of this illness, including an exceptionally high death rate for young adults aged between 20 and 40 years.

In contrast to the Spanish flu, coronavirus is not so common, has caused in fewer fatalities, has a higher case fatality rate, is more harmful to older ages and is less risky for individuals aged 20–40 years.

1.2.9 Coronavirus Versus Common Cold (Typically Rhinovirus)

Common cold is the most common illness impacting people—Typically, a person suffers from 2–3 colds each year and the average kid will catch 6–8 during the similar time span. Although there are more than 200 cold-associated virus types, infections are uncommon and fatalities are very rare and typically arise mainly in extremely old, extremely young or immunosuppressed cases [43, 44].

In contrast to the common cold, coronavirus is not so prevalent, causes more fatalities, has more case fatality rate, is less infectious and is less likely to impact small children.

1.3   Reviews of Online Portals and Social Media for Epidemic Information Dissemination

As COVID-19 started to propagate across the globe, the outbreak contributed to a significant change in the broad technology platforms. Where they once declined to engage in the affairs of their systems, except though the possible danger to public safety became obvious, the advent of a novel coronavirus placed them in a different interventionist way of thought. Big tech firms and social media are taking concrete steps to guide users to relevant, credible details on the virus [45–48]. And some of the measures they're doing proactively. Below are a few of them.

Facebook started adding a box in the news feed that led users to the Centers for Disease Control website regarding COVID-19. It reflects a significant departure from the company's normal strategy of placing items in the News Feed. The purpose of the update, after all, is personalization—Facebook tries to give the posts you're going to care about, whether it is because you're connected with a person or like a post. In the virus package, Facebook has placed a remarkable algorithmic thumb on the scale, potentially pushing millions of people to accurate, authenticated knowledge from a reputable source.

Similar initiatives have been adopted by Twitter. Searching for COVID-19 will carry you to a page highlighting the latest reports from public health groups and credible national news outlets. The search also allows for common misspellings. Twitter has stated that although Russian-style initiatives to cause discontent by large-scale intelligence operations have not yet been observed, a zero-tolerance approach to network exploitation and all other attempts to exploit their service at this crucial juncture will be expected. The problem has the attention of the organization. It also offers promotional support to public service agencies and other non-profit groups.

Google has made a step in making it better for those who choose to operate or research from home, offering specialized streaming services to all paying G Suite customers. Google also confirmed that free access to 'advanced' Hangouts Meet apps will be rolled out to both G Suite and G Suite for Education clients worldwide through 1st July. It ensures that companies can hold meetings of up to 250 people, broadcast live to up to about 100,000 users within a single network, and archive and export meetings to Google Drive. Usually, Google pays an additional $13 per person per month for these services in comparison to G Suite's 'enterprise' membership, which adds up to a total of about $25 per client each month.

Microsoft took a similar move, introducing the software 'Chat Device' to help public health and protection in the coronavirus epidemic, which enables collaborative collaboration via video and text messaging. There's an aspect of self-interest in this. Tech firms are offering out their goods free of charge during periods of emergency for the same purpose as newspapers are reducing their paywalls: it's nice to draw more paying consumers.

Pinterest, which has introduced much of the anti-misinformation strategies that Facebook and Twitter are already embracing, is now restricting the search results for 'coronavirus', 'COVID-19' and similar words for 'internationally recognized health organizations'.

Google-owned YouTube, traditionally the most conspiratorial website, has recently introduced a connection to the World Health Organization virus epidemic page to the top of the search results. In the early days of the epidemic, BuzzFeed found famous coronavirus conspiratorial videos on YouTube—especially in India, where one 'explain' with a false interpretation of the sources of the disease racketeered 13 million views before YouTube deleted it. Yet in the United States, conspiratorial posts regarding the illness have failed to gain only 1 million views.

That's not to suggest that misinformation doesn't propagate on digital platforms—just as it travels through the broader Internet, even though interaction with friends and relatives. When there's a site that appears to be under-performing in the global epidemic, it's Facebook-owned WhatsApp, where the Washington Post reported 'a torrent of disinformation' in places like Nigeria, Indonesia, Peru, Pakistan and Ireland. Given the encrypted existence of the app, it is difficult to measure the severity of the problem. Misinformation is also spread in WhatsApp communities, where participation is restricted to about 250 individuals. Knowledge of one category may be readily exchanged with another; however, there is a considerable amount of complexity of rotating several groups to peddle affected healing remedies or propagate false rumours.

1.4 Preventative Measures and Policies Enforced by the World Health Organization (WHO) and Different Countries

Coronavirus is already an ongoing epidemic, so it is necessary to take precautions to minimize both the risk of being sick and the transmission of the disease.

1.4.1 WHO Advice [49]

- Wash hands regularly with alcohol-based hand wash or soap and water.
- Preserve contact space (at least 1 m/3 feet between you and someone who sneezes or coughs).
- Don't touch your nose, head and ears.
- Cover your nose and mouth as you sneeze or cough, preferably with your bent elbow or tissue.
- Try to find early medical attention if you have fatigue, cough and trouble breathing.
- Take preventive precautions if you are in or have recently go to places where coronavirus spreads.

1.4.2   China

The first person believed to have become sick because of the latest virus was near in Wuhan on 1 December 2019. A formal warning of the epidemic was released on 31 December. The World Health Organization was informed of the epidemic on the same day. Through 7 January, the Chinese Government addressed the avoidance and regulation of COVID-19. A curfew was declared on 23 January to prohibit flying in and out of Wuhan. Private usage of cars has been banned in the region. Chinese New Year (25 January) festivities have been cancelled in many locations [50].

On 26 January, the Communist Party and the Government adopted more steps to contain the COVID-19 epidemic, including safety warnings for travellers and improvements to national holidays. The leading party has agreed to prolong the Spring Festival holiday to control the outbreak. Universities and schools across the world have already been locked down. Many steps have been taken by the Hong Kong and Macau governments, in particular concerning schools and colleges. Remote job initiatives have been placed in effect in many regions of China. Several immigration limits have been enforced.

Certain counties and cities outside Hubei also implemented travel limits. Public transit has been changed and museums in China have been partially removed. Some experts challenged the quality of the number of cases announced by the Chinese Government, which constantly modified the way coronavirus cases were recorded.

1.4.3   Italy

Italy, a member state of the European Union and a popular tourist attraction, entered the list of coronavirus-affected nations on 30 January, when two positive cases in COVID-19 were identified among Chinese tourists. Italy has the largest number of coronavirus infections both in Europe and outside of China [51].

Infections, originally limited to northern Italy, gradually spread to all other areas. Many other nations in Asia, Europe and the Americas have tracked their local cases to Italy. Several Italian travellers were even infected with coronavirus-positive in foreign nations.

Late in Italy, the most impacted coronavirus cities and counties are Lombardia, accompanied by Veneto, Emilia-Romagna, Marche and Piedmonte. Milan, the second most populated city in Italy, is situated in Lombardy. Other regions in Italy with coronavirus comprised Campania, Toscana, Liguria, Lazio, Sicilia, Friuli Venezia Giulia, Umbria, Puglia, Trento, Abruzzo, Calabria, Molise, Valle d'Aosta, Sardegna, Bolzano and Basilicata.

Italy ranks 19th of the top 30 nations getting high-risk coronavirus airline passengers in China, as per WorldPop's provisional study of the spread of COVID-19.

The Italian State has taken steps like the inspection and termination of large cultural activities during the early days of the coronavirus epidemic and has gradually declared the closing of educational establishments and airport hygiene/disinfection initiatives.

The Italian National Institute of Health suggested social distancing and agreed that the broader community of the country's elderly is a problem. In the meantime, several other nations, including the US, have recommended that travel to Italy should be avoided temporarily, unless necessary.

The Italian government has declared the closing (quarantine) of the impacted areas in the northern region of the nation so as not to spread to the rest of the world. Italy has declared the immediate suspension of all to-and-fro air travel with China following coronavirus discovery by a Chinese tourist to Italy. Italian airlines, like Ryan Air, have begun introducing protective steps and have begun calling for the declaration forms to be submitted by passengers flying to Poland, Slovakia and Lithuania.

The Italian government first declined to permit fans to compete in sporting activities until early April to prevent the potential transmission of coronavirus. The step ensured players of health and stopped event cancellations because of coronavirus fears. Two days of the declaration, the government cancelled all athletic activities owing to the emergence of the outbreak asking for an emergency. Sports activities in Veneto, Lombardy and Emilia-Romagna, which recorded coronavirus-positive infections, were confirmed to be temporarily suspended. Schools and colleges in Italy have also been forced to shut down.

1.4.4   Iran

Iran announced the first recorded cases of SARS-CoV-2 infection on 19 February when, as per the Medical Education and Ministry of Health, two persons died later that day. The Ministry of Islamic Culture and Guidance has declared the cancellation of all concerts and other cultural activities for one week. The Medical Education and Ministry of Health has also declared the closing of universities, higher education colleges and schools in many cities and regions. The Department of Sports and Culture has taken action to suspend athletic activities, including football matches [52].

On 2 March 2020, the government revealed plans to train about 300,000 troops and volunteers to fight the outbreak of the epidemic, and also send robots and water cannons to clean the cities. The State also developed an initiative and a webpage to counter the epidemic. On 9 March 2020, nearly 70,000 inmates were immediately released from jail owing to the epidemic, presumably to prevent the further dissemination of the disease inside jails. The Revolutionary Guards declared a campaign on 13 March 2020 to clear highways, stores and public areas in Iran. President Hassan Rouhani stated on 26 February 2020 that there were no arrangements to quarantine areas impacted by the epidemic and only persons should be quarantined. The temples of Shia in Qom stayed open to pilgrims.

1.4.5   South Korea

On 20 January, South Korea announced its first occurrence. There was a large rise in cases on 20 February, possibly due to the meeting in Daegu of a progressive faith community recognized as the Shincheonji Church of Christ. Any citizens believed that the hospital was propagating the disease. As of 22 February, 1,261 of the 9,336 members of the church registered symptoms. A petition was distributed calling for the abolition of the church. More than 2,000 verified cases were registered on 28 February, increasing to 3,150 on 29 February [53].

Several educational establishments have been partially closing down, including hundreds of kindergartens in Daegu and many primary schools in Seoul. As of 18 February, several South Korean colleges had confirmed intentions to delay the launch of the spring semester. That included 155 institutions deciding to postpone the start of the semester by two weeks until 16 March, and 22 institutions deciding to delay the start of the semester by one week until 9 March. Also, on 23 February 2020, all primary schools, kindergartens, middle schools and secondary schools were declared to postpone the start of the semester from 2 March to 9 March.

South Korea's economy is expected to expand by 1.9%, down from 2.1%. The State has given 136.7 billion won funding to local councils. The State has also coordinated the purchase of masks and other sanitary supplies. Entertainment Company SM Entertainment is confirmed to have contributed five hundred million won in attempts to fight the disease.

In the kpop industry, the widespread dissemination of coronavirus within South Korea has contributed to the cancellation or postponement of concerts and other programmes for kpop activities inside and outside South Korea. For instance, circumstances such as the cancellation of the remaining Asian dates and the European leg for the Seventeen's Ode To You Tour on 9 February 2020 and the cancellation of all Seoul dates for the BTS Soul Tour Map. As of 15 March, a maximum of 136 countries and regions provided entry restrictions and/or expired visas for passengers from South Korea.

1.4.6   France

The overall reported cases of coronavirus rose significantly in France on 12 March. The areas with reported cases include Paris, Amiens, Bordeaux and Eastern Haute-Savoie. The first coronaviral death happened in France on 15 February, marking it the first death in Europe. The second death of a 60-year-old French national in Paris was announced on 26 February [54].

On February 28, fashion designer Agnès B. (not to be mistaken with Agnès Buzyn) cancelled fashion shows at the Paris Fashion Week, expected to continue until 3 March. On a subsequent day, the Paris half-marathon, planned for Sunday 1 March with 44,000 entrants, was postponed as one of a series of steps declared by Health Minister Olivier Véran.

On 13 March, the Ligue de Football Professional disbanded Ligue 1 and Ligue 2 (France's tier two professional divisions) permanently due to safety threats.

1.4.7 Germany

Germany has a popular Regional Pandemic Strategy detailing the roles and activities of the health care system participants in the case of a significant outbreak. Epidemic surveillance is carried out by the federal government, like the Robert Koch Center, and by the German governments. The German States have their preparations for an outbreak. The regional strategy for the treatment of the current coronavirus epidemic was expanded by March 2020. Four primary goals are contained in this plan: (1) to minimize mortality and morbidity; (2) to guarantee the safety of sick persons; (3) to protect vital health services and (4) to offer concise and reliable reports to decision-makers, the media and the public [55].

The programme has three phases that may potentially overlap: (1) isolation (situation of individual cases and clusters), (2) safety (situation of further dissemination of pathogens and suspected causes of infection), (3) prevention (situation of widespread infection). So far, Germany has not set up border controls or common health condition tests at airports. Instead, while at the isolation stage-health officials are concentrating on recognizing contact individuals that are subject to specific quarantine and are tracked and checked. Specific quarantine is regulated by municipal health authorities. By doing so, the officials are seeking to hold the chains of infection small, contributing to decreased clusters. At the safety stage, the policy should shift to prevent susceptible individuals from being harmed by direct action. By the end of the day, the prevention process should aim to prevent cycles of acute treatment to retain emergency facilities.

1.4.8 United States

The very first case of coronavirus in the United States was identified in Washington on 21 January 2020 by an individual who flew to Wuhan and returned to the United States. The second case was recorded in Illinois by another individual who had travelled to Wuhan. Some of the regions with reported novel coronavirus infections in the US are California, Arizona, Connecticut, Illinois, Texas, Wisconsin and Washington [56].

As the epidemic increased, requests for domestic air travel decreased dramatically. By 4 March, U.S. carriers, like United Airlines and JetBlue Airways, started growing their domestic flight schedules, providing generous unpaid leave to workers and suspending recruits.

A significant number of universities and colleges cancelled classes and reopened dormitories in response to the epidemic, like Cornell University, Harvard University and the University of South Carolina.

On 3 March 2020, the Federal Reserve reduced its goal interest rate from 1.75% to 1.25%, the biggest emergency rate cut following the 2008 global financial crash, in combat the effect of the recession on the American economy. In February 2020, US businesses, including Apple Inc. and Microsoft, started to reduce sales projections due to supply chain delays in China caused by the COVID-19.

The pandemic, together with the subsequent financial market collapse, also contributed to greater criticism of the crisis in the United States. Researchers disagree about when a recession is likely to take effect, with others suggesting that it is not unavoidable, while some claim that the world might already be in recession. On 3 March, Federal Reserve Chairman Jerome Powell reported a 0.5% (50 basis point) interest rate cut from the coronavirus in the context of the evolving threats to economic growth.

When 'social distance' penetrated the national lexicon, disaster response officials promoted the cancellation of broad events to slow down the risk of infection. Technical conferences like E3 2020, Apple Inc.'s Worldwide Developers Conference (WWDC), Google I/O, Facebook F8, and Cloud Next and Microsoft's MVP Conference have been either having replaced or cancelled in-person events with internet streaming events.

On February 29, the American Physical Society postponed its annual March gathering, planned for March 2–6 in Denver, Colorado, even though most of the more than 11,000 physicist attendees already had arrived and engaged in the pre-conference day activities. On March 6, the annual South to Southwest (SXSW) seminar and festival planned to take place from March 13–22 in Austin, Texas, was postponed after the city council announced a local disaster and forced conferences to be shut down for the first time in 34 years.

Four of North America's major professional sports leagues—the National Hockey League (NHL), National Basketball Association (NBA), Major League Soccer (MLS) and Major League Baseball (MLB) —jointly declared on March 9 that they would all limit the media access to player accommodations (such as locker rooms) to control probable exposure.

1.5 Emergency Funding to Fight the COVID-19

COVID-19 pandemic has become a common international concern. Different countries are donating funds to fight against it [57–60]. Some of them are mentioned here.

China has allocated about 110.48 billion yuan ($15.93 billion) in coronavirus-related funding.

Foreign Minister Mohammad Javad Zarif said that Iran has requested the International Monetary Fund (IMF) of about $5 billion in emergency funding to help to tackle the coronavirus epidemic that has struck the Islamic Republic hard.

President Donald Trump approved the Emergency Supplementary Budget Bill to support the US response to a novel coronavirus epidemic. The budget plan would include about $8.3 billion in discretionary funding to local health authorities to promote vaccine research for production. Trump originally requested just about $2 billion to combat the epidemic, but Congress quadrupled the number in its version of the bill. Mr. Trump formally announced a national emergency that he claimed it will give states and territories access to up to about $50 billion in federal funding to tackle the spread of the coronavirus outbreak.

California politicians approved a plan to donate about $1 billion on the state's emergency medical responses as it readies hospitals to fight an expected attack of patients because of the COVID-19 pandemic. The plans, drawn up rapidly in reaction to the dramatic rise in reported cases of the virus, would include the requisite funds to establish two new hospitals in California, with the assumption that the state may not have the resources to take care of the rise in patients. The bill calls for an immediate response of about $500 million from the State General Fund, with an additional about $500 million possible if requested.

India committed about $10 million to the COVID-19 Emergency Fund and said it was setting up a rapid response team of physicians for the South Asian Association for Regional Cooperation (Saarc) countries.

South Korea unveiled an economic stimulus package of about 11.7 trillion won ($9.8 billion) to soften the effects of the biggest coronavirus epidemic outside China as attempts to curb the disease exacerbate supply shortages and drain demand. Of the 11,7 trillion won expected, about 3.2 trillion won would cover up the budget shortfall, while an additional fiscal infusion of about 8.5 trillion won. An estimated 10.3 trillion won in government bonds will be sold this year to fund the extra expenditure. About 2.3 trillion won will be distributed to medical establishments and would support quarantine operations, with another 3.0 trillion won heading to small and medium-sized companies unable to pay salaries to their employees and child care supports.

The Swedish Parliament announced a set of initiatives costing more than 300 billion Swedish crowns ($30.94 billion) to help the economy in the view of the coronavirus pandemic. The plan contained steps like the central government paying the entire expense of the company's sick leave during April and May, and also the high cost of compulsory redundancies owing to the crisis.

In consideration of the developing scenario, an updating of this strategy is planned to take place before the end of March and will recognize considerably greater funding demands for the country response, R&D and WHO itself.

1.6 Artificial Intelligence, Data Science and Technological Solutions Against COVID-19

These days, Artificial Intelligence (AI) takes a major role in health care. Throughout a worldwide pandemic such as the COVID-19, technology, artificial intelligence and data analytics have been crucial in helping communities cope successfully with the epidemic [61–65]. Through the aid of data mining and analytical modelling, medical practitioners are willing to learn more about several diseases.

1.6.1 Public Health Surveillance

The biggest risk of coronavirus is the level of spreading. That's why policymakers are introducing steps like quarantines around the world because they can't adequately monitor local outbreaks. One of the simplest measures to identify ill patients through the study of CCTV images that are still around us and to locate and separate individuals that have serious signs of the disease and who have touched and disinfected the related surfaces. Smartphone applications are often used to keep a watch on people's activities and to assess whether or not they have come in touch with an infected human.

1.6.2 Remote Biosignal Measurement

Many of the signs such as temperature or heartbeat are very essential to overlook and rely entirely on the visual image that may be misleading. However, of course, we can't prevent someone from checking their blood pressure, heart or temperature. Also, several advances in computer vision can predict pulse and blood pressure based on facial skin examination. Besides, there are several advances in computer vision that can predict pulse and blood pressure based on facial skin examination.

Access to public records has contributed to the development of dashboards that constantly track the virus. Several companies are designing large data dashboards. Face recognition and infrared temperature monitoring technologies have been mounted in all major cities. Chinese AI companies including Hanwang Technology and SenseTime have reported having established a special facial recognition system that can correctly identify people even though they are covered.

1.6.3 IoT and Wearables

Measurements like pulse are much more natural and easier to obtain from tracking gadgets like activity trackers and smartwatches that nearly everybody has already. Some work suggests that the study of cardiac activity and its variations from the standard will reveal early signs of influenza and, in this case, coronavirus.

1.6.4 Chatbots and Communication

Apart from public screening, people's knowledge and self-assessment may also be used to track their health. If you can check your temperature and pulse every day and monitor your coughs time-to-time, you can even submit that to your record. If the symptoms are too serious, either an algorithm or a doctor remotely may prescribe a person to stay home, take several other preventive measures, or recommend a visit from the doctor.

Al Jazeera announced that China Mobile had sent text messages to state media departments, telling them about the citizens who had been affected. The communications contained all the specifics of the person's travel history.

Tencent runs WeChat, and via it, citizens can use free online health consultation services. Chatbots have already become important connectivity platforms for transport and tourism service providers to keep passengers up-to-date with the current transport protocols and disturbances.

1.6.5 Social Media and Open Data

There are several people who post their health diary with total strangers via Facebook or Twitter. Such data becomes helpful for more general research about how far the epidemic has progressed. For consumer knowledge, we may even evaluate the social network group to attempt to predict what specific networks are at risk of being viral.

Canadian company BlueDot analyses far more than just social network data: for instance, global activities of more than four billion passengers on international flights per year; animal, human and insect population data; satellite environment data and relevant knowledge from health professionals and journalists, across 100,000 news posts per day covering 65 languages. This strategy was so successful that the corporation was able to alert clients about coronavirus until the World Health Organization and the Centers for Disease Control and Prevention notified the public.

1.6.6 Automated Diagnostics

COVID-19 has brought up another healthcare issue today: it will not scale when the number of patients increases exponentially (actually stressed doctors are always doing worse) and the rate of false-negative diagnosis remains very high. Machine learning therapies don't get bored and scale simply by growing computing forces.

Baidu, the Chinese Internet company, has made the Lineatrfold algorithm accessible to the outbreak-fighting teams, according to the MIT Technology Review. Unlike HIV, Ebola and Influenza, COVID-19 has just one strand of RNA and it can mutate easily. The algorithm is also simpler than other algorithms that help to determine the nature of the virus. Baidu has also developed software to efficiently track large populations. It has also developed an Ai-powered infrared device that can detect a difference in the body temperature of a human. This is currently being used in Beijing's Qinghe Railway Station to classify possibly contaminated travellers where up to 200 individuals may be checked in one minute without affecting traffic movement, reports the MIT Review.

Singapore-based Veredus Laboratories, a supplier of revolutionary molecular diagnostic tools, has currently announced the launch of the VereCoV detector package, a compact Lab-on-Chip device able to detect MERS-CoV, SARS-CoV and COVID-19, i.e. Wuhan Coronavirus, in a single study.

The VereCoV identification package is focused on VereChip technology, a Lab-on-Chip device that incorporates two important molecular biological systems, Polymerase Chain Reaction (PCR) and a microarray, which will be able to classify and distinguish within 2 h MERS-CoV, SARS-CoV and COVID-19 with high precision and responsiveness.

This is not just the medical activities of healthcare facilities that are being charged, but also the corporate and financial departments when they cope with the increase in patients. Ant Financials' blockchain technology helps speed-up the collection of reports and decreases the number of face-to-face encounters with patients and medical personnel.

Companies like the Israeli company Sonovia are aiming to provide healthcare systems and others with face masks manufactured from their anti-pathogenic, anti-bacterial cloth that depends on metal-oxide nanoparticles.

1.6.7 Drug Development Research

Aside from identifying and stopping the transmission of pathogens, the need to develop vaccinations on a scale is also needed. One of the crucial things to make that possible is to consider the origin and essence of the virus. Google's DeepMind, with their expertise in protein folding research, has rendered a jump in identifying the protein structure of the virus and making it open-source.

BenevolentAI uses AI technologies to develop medicines that will combat the most dangerous diseases in the world and is also working to promote attempts to cure coronavirus, the first time the organization has based its product on infectious diseases. Within weeks of the epidemic, it used its analytical capability to recommend new medicines that might be beneficial.

1.6.8 Robotics

Robots are not vulnerable to the infection, and they are used to conduct other activities, like cooking meals in hospitals, doubling up as waiters in hotels, spraying disinfectants and washing, selling rice and hand sanitizers, robots are on the front lines all over to deter coronavirus spread. Robots also conduct diagnostics and thermal imaging in several hospitals. Shenzhen-based firm Multicopter uses robotics to move surgical samples. UVD robots from Blue Ocean Robotics use ultraviolet light to destroy viruses and bacteria separately. In China, Pudu Technology has introduced its robots, which are usually used in the cooking industry, to more than 40 hospitals throughout the region. According to the Reuters article, a tiny robot named Little Peanut is distributing food to passengers who have been on a flight from Singapore to Hangzhou, China, and are presently being quarantined in a hotel.

1.6.9 Colour Coding

Using its advanced and vast public service monitoring network, the Chinese government has collaborated with software companies Alibaba and Tencent to establish a colour-coded health ranking scheme that monitors millions of citizens every day. The mobile device was first introduced in Hangzhou with the cooperation of Alibaba. This applies three colours to people—red, green or yellow—based on their transportation and medical records. Tencent also developed related applications in the manufacturing centre of Shenzhen.

The decision of whether an individual will be quarantined or permitted in public spaces is dependent on the colour code. Citizens will sign into the system using pay wallet systems such as Alibaba's Alipay and Ant's wallet. Just those citizens who have been issued a green colour code will be permitted to use the QR code in public spaces at metro stations, workplaces, and other public areas. Checkpoints are in most public areas where the body temperature and the code of individual are tested. This programme is being used by more than 200 Chinese communities and will eventually be expanded nationwide.

1.6.10 Drones

In some of the seriously infected regions where people remain at risk of contracting the infection, drones are used to rescue. One of the easiest and quickest ways to bring emergency supplies where they need to go while on an epidemic of disease is by drone transportation. Drones carry all surgical instruments and patient samples. This saves time, improves the pace of distribution and reduces the chance of contamination of medical samples. Drones often operate QR code placards that can be checked to record health records. There are also agricultural drones distributing disinfectants in the farmland. Drones, operated by facial recognition, are often used to warn people not to leave their homes and to chide them for not using face masks. Terra Drone uses its unmanned drones to move patient samples and vaccination content at reduced risk between the Xinchang County Disease Control Center and the People's Hospital. Drones are often used to monitor public areas, document non-compliance with quarantine laws and thermal imaging.

1.6.11 Autonomous Vehicles

At a period of considerable uncertainty to medical professionals and the danger to people-to-people communication, automated vehicles are proving to be of tremendous benefit in the transport of vital products, such as medications and foodstuffs. Apollo, the Baidu Autonomous Vehicle Project, has joined hands with the Neolix self-driving company to distribute food and supplies to a big hospital in Beijing. Baidu Apollo has also provided its micro-car packages and automated cloud driving systems accessible free of charge to virus-fighting organizations.

Idriverplus, a Chinese self-driving organization that runs electrical street cleaning vehicles, is also part of the project. The company's signature trucks are used to clean hospitals.

1.7 Summary

This chapter provides an introduction to the coronavirus outbreak (COVID-19). A brief history of this virus along with the symptoms are reported in this chapter. Then the comparison between COVID-19 and other plagues like seasonal influenza, bird flu (H5N1 and H7N9), Ebola epidemic, camel flu (MERS), swine flu (H1N1), severe acute respiratory syndrome, Hong Kong flu (H3N2), Spanish flu and the common cold are included in this chapter. Reviews of online portal and social media like Facebook, Twitter, Google, Microsoft, Pinterest, YouTube and WhatsApp concerning COVID-19 are reported in this chapter. Also, the preventive measures and policies enforced by WHO and different countries such as China, Italy, Iran, South Korea, France,

Germany and the United States for COVID-19 are included in this chapter. Emergency funding provided by different countries to fight the COVID-19 is mentioned in this chapter. Lastly, artificial intelligence, data science and technological solutions like public health surveillance, remote biosignal measurement, IoT and wearables, chatbots and communication, social media and open data, automated diagnostics, drug development research, robotics, colour coding, drones and autonomous vehicles are included in this chapter.

References

1. Hui DS et al (2020) The continuing 2019-nCoV epidemic threat of novel coronaviruses to global health—the latest 2019 novel coronavirus outbreak in Wuhan, China. Inte J Infectious Dis 91:264–266
2. Read JM, Bridgen JR, Cummings DA, Ho A, Jewell CP (2020) Novel coronavirus 2019-nCoV: early estimation of epidemiological parameters and epidemic predictions. *medRxiv*
3. Corman VM et al (2020) Detection of 2019 novel coronavirus (2019-nCoV) by real-time RT-PCR. Eurosurveillance 25(3)
4. Fong SJ, Li G, Dey N, Crespo RG, Herrera-Viedma E (2020) composite monte carlo decision making under high uncertainty of novel coronavirus epidemic using hybridized deep learning and fuzzy rule induction. arXiv preprint arXiv:2003.09868
5. China just banned the trade and consumption of wild animals. Experts think the coronavirus jumped from live animals to people at a market. https://www.businessinsider.in/science/news/china-just-banned-the-trade-and-consumption-of-wild-animals-experts-think-the-cor onavirus-jumped-from-live-animals-to-people-at-a-market-/articleshow/74309474.cms
6. Calls for global ban on wild animal markets amid coronavirus outbreak https://www.thegua rdian.com/science/2020/jan/24/calls-for-global-ban-on-wild-animal-markets-amid-coronavirus-outbreak
7. Coronavirus closures reveal vast scale of China's secretive wildlife farm https://www.thegua rdian.com/environment/2020/feb/25/coronavirus-closures-reveal-vast-scale-of-chinas-secret ive-wildlife-farm-industry
8. Chinese citizens push to abolish wildlife trade as coronavirus persists https://www.nationalg eographic.com/animals/2020/01/china-bans-wildlife-trade-after-coronavirus-outbreak/
9. Woo PC et al (2012) Discovery of seven novel Mammalian and avian coronaviruses in the genus deltacoronavirus supports bat coronaviruses as the gene source of alphacoronavirus and betacoronavirus and avian coronaviruses as the gene source of gammacoronavirus and deltacoronavirus. J Virol 86(7):3995–4008
10. Fong SJ, Li G, Dey N, Crespo RG, Herrera-Viedma E (2020) Finding an accurate early forecasting model from small dataset: a case of 2019-ncov novel coronavirus outbreak. arXiv preprint arXiv:2003.10776
11. Ge XY et al (2017) Detection of alpha-and betacoronaviruses in rodents from Yunnan China. Virol J 14(1):98
12. Can We Learn Anything from the SARS Outbreak to Fight COVID-19? https://www.health line.com/health-news/has-anything-changed-since-the-2003-sars-outbreak
13. Huang Y (2004) The SARS epidemic and its aftermath in China: a political perspective. Learning from SARS: Preparing for the next disease outbreak, 116–36
14. Hung LS (2003) The SARS epidemic in Hong Kong: what lessons have we learned? J R Soc Med 96(8):374–378
15. Rajinikanth V, Dey N, Raj ANJ, Hassanien AE, Santosh KC, Raja N (2020) Harmony-search and Otsu based system for coronavirus disease (COVID-19) detection using Lung CT scan images. arXiv preprint arXiv:2004.03431

16. Kim KH, Tandi TE, Choi JW, Moon JM, Kim MS (2017) Middle East respiratory syndrome coronavirus (MERS-CoV) outbreak in South Korea, 2015: epidemiology, characteristics and public health implications. J Hosp Infect 95(2):207–213

17. Sikkema RS, Farag EABA, Islam M, Atta M, Reusken CBEM, Al-Hajri MM, Koopmans MPG (2019) Global status of Middle East respiratory syndrome coronavirus in dromedary camels: a systematic review. Epidemiol Infect, 147

18. Wickramasinghe NC et al (2020) Comments on the origin and spread of the 2019 Coronavirus. Virol Curr Res 4(1)

19. Sun Z, Xu P, Liu X, Karuppiah T, Kumar SS, He G (2020) A Review on the factors contributing to 2019-nCoV virus outbreaks in Wuhan

20. Dietz L, Horve PF, Coil D, Fretz M, Van Den Wymelenberg K (2020) 2019 Novel Coronavirus (COVID-19) outbreak: a review of the current literature and built environment (BE) considerations to reduce transmission

21. How does the new coronavirus compare with the flu? https://www.livescience.com/new-coronavirus-compare-with-flu.html

22. Coronavirus vs. Flu: Which Virus Is Deadlier? https://www.wsj.com/articles/coronavirus-vs-flu-which-virus-is-deadlier-11583856879

23. Coronavirus vs. the Flu: The Difference Between a 1% and 0.1% Fatality Rate Is Huge https://www.nationalreview.com/corner/coronavirus-vs-the-flu-the-difference-between-a-1-and-0-1-fatality-rate-is-huge/

24. How Does the New Coronavirus Compare with the Flu? https://www.scientificamerican.com/article/how-does-the-new-coronavirus-compare-with-the-flu/

25. China hit by second deadly virus as bird flu strikes near coronavirus city https://metro.co.uk/2020/02/02/china-hit-by-second-deadly-virus-as-bird-flu-strikes-near-coronavirus-city-12168549/

26. Fatality rate of major virus outbreaks worldwide in the last 50 years as of 2020 https://www.statista.com/statistics/1095129/worldwide-fatality-rate-of-major-virus-outbreaks-in-the-last-50-years/

27. Here's How COVID-19 Compares to Past Outbreaks https://www.healthline.com/health-news/how-deadly-is-the-coronavirus-compared-to-past-outbreaks

28. Coronavirus: The lessons to learn from Ebola https://www.dw.com/en/coronavirus-the-lessons-to-learn-from-ebola/a-52759301

29. Lessons from an Ebola survivor: Here's what we can do about the coronavirus https://www.bostonglobe.com/2020/03/16/magazine/i-survived-ebola-well-make-it-through-coronavirus-too/

30. Middle East respiratory syndrome coronavirus (MERS-CoV) https://www.who.int/news-room/fact-sheets/detail/middle-east-respiratory-syndrome-coronavirus-(mers-cov)

31. Deadly MERS 'camel flu' may now be airborne https://www.nhs.uk/news/medical-practice/deadly-mers-camel-flu-may-now-be-airborne/

32. Bhatia PK, Sethi P, Gupta N, Biyani G (2016) Middle East respiratory syndrome: a new global threat. Indian J Anaesthesia 60(2):85

33. Coronavirus vs. Swine Flu—the numbers https://upnorthlive.com/news/local/coronavirus-vs-swine-flu-the-numbers

34. How the coronavirus compares to SARS, swine flu, Zika, and other epidemics https://www.businessinsider.in/international/news/how-the-coronavirus-compares-to-sars-swine-flu-zika-and-other-epidemics/articleshow/74560116.cms

35. Swine flu and coronavirus: Are these pandemics different? https://www.wkrn.com/news/swine-flu-and-coronavirus-are-these-pandemics-different/

36. Ghinai I et al (2020) First known person-to-person transmission of severe acute respiratory syndrome coronavirus 2 (SARS-CoV-2) in the USA. The Lancet

37. Scientists Compare Novel Coronavirus with SARS and MERS Viruses https://www.the-scientist.com/news-opinion/scientists-compare-novel-coronavirus-to-sars-and-mers-viruses-67088

38. Coronaviruses https://www.niaid.nih.gov/diseases-conditions/coronaviruses

39. Closed borders and 'black weddings': what the 1918 flu teaches us about coronavirus https://www.theguardian.com/world/2020/mar/11/closed-borders-and-black-weddings-what-the-1918-flu-teaches-us-about-coronavirus

40. Rampant Lies, Fake Cures and Not Enough Beds: What the Spanish Flu Debacle Can Teach Us About Coronavirus https://www.politico.com/news/magazine/2020/03/17/spanish-flu-lessons-coronavirus-133888
41. Why we should stop comparing the Covid-19 coronavirus outbreak to the 1918 Spanish flu https://www.vox.com/2020/3/9/21164957/covid-19-spanish-flu-mortality-rate-death-rate
42. Coronavirus pandemic vs. Spanish flu! Then and now https://www.cantonrep.com/news/20200315/coronavirus-pandemic-vs-spanish-flu–then-and-now
43. What's the difference between a cold, the flu, and coronavirus? https://intermountainhealthcare.org/blogs/topics/live-well/2020/03/whats-the-difference-between-a-cold-the-flu-and-coronavirus/
44. Not Sure You Have COVID-19? Here Are the Symptoms for Coronavirus, Flu, and Allergies https://www.healthline.com/health-news/flu-allergies-coronavirus-different-symptoms
45. Here's how social media can combat the coronavirus 'infodemic' https://www.technologyreview.com/s/615368/facebook-twitter-social-media-infodemic-misinformation/
46. Coronavirus may affect your social media. https://www.indiatoday.in/world/story/coronavirus-may-affect-your-social-media-read-how-1656306-2020-03-17
47. How Social Media Is Shaping Our Fears of—and Response to—the Coronavirus https://time.com/5802802/social-media-coronavirus/
48. Social media firms will use more AI to combat coronavirus misinformation, even if it makes more mistakes https://thenextweb.com/neural/2020/03/17/social-media-firms-will-use-more-ai-to-combat-coronavirus-misinformation-even-if-it-makes-more-mistakes/
49. Coronavirus disease (COVID-19) technical guidance: Infection prevention and control/WASH https://www.who.int/emergencies/diseases/novel-coronavirus-2019/technical-guidance/infection-prevention-and-control
50. extreme measures China took to contain the coronavirus show the rest of the world is unprepared for COVID-19 https://www.businessinsider.in/science/news/11-extreme-measures-china-took-to-contain-the-coronavirus-show-the-rest-of-the-world-is-unprepared-for-covid-19/articleshow/74660747.cms
51. Coronavirus in Italy: Outbreak, measures and impact https://www.pharmaceutical-technology.com/features/covid-19-italy-coronavirus-deaths-measures-airports-tourism/
52. Iran reports its largest coronavirus death toll within 24-hour period https://www.france24.com/en/20200308-iran-reports-its-largest-coronavirus-death-toll-within-24-hour-period
53. Coronavirus in South Korea: Covid-19 outbreak, measures and impact https://www.pharmaceutical-technology.com/features/coronavirus-affected-countries-south-korea-covid-19-outbreak-measures-impact/
54. Spain, France take drastic measures to fight coronavirus; Georgia delays presidential primary https://www.washingtonpost.com/world/2020/03/14/coronavirus-latest-news/
55. Coronavirus: These are the measures in Germany you need to know about https://www.thelocal.de/20200313/coronavirus-these-are-the-measures-germany-is-asking-you-to-take
56. How to prepare for coronavirus in the U.S. https://www.washingtonpost.com/health/2020/02/26/how-to-prepare-for-coronavirus/?arc404=true
57. Contributions to WHO for COVID-19 appeal https://www.who.int/emergencies/diseases/novel-coronavirus-2019/donors-and-partners/funding
58. Coronavirus: EU mobilises €10 million for research https://ec.europa.eu/info/news/coronavirus-eu-mobilises-eur10-million-for-research-2020-jan-31_en
59. COVID-19—a timeline of the coronavirus outbreak https://www.devex.com/news/covid-19-a-timeline-of-the-coronavirus-outbreak-96396
60. Coronavirus global health emergency: Coverage from UN News https://news.un.org/en/node/1039401/date/2020-03-01
61. Coronavirus: How Artificial Intelligence, Data Science And Technology Is Used To Fight The Pandemic https://www.forbes.com/sites/bernardmarr/2020/03/13/coronavirus-how-artificial-intelligence-data-science-and-technology-is-used-to-fight-the-pandemic/#520062fe5f5f
62. Researchers Will Deploy AI to Better Understand Coronavirus https://www.wired.com/story/researchers-deploy-ai-better-understand-coronavirus/

63. How A.I. is aiding the coronavirus fight https://fortune.com/2020/03/16/ai-coronavirus-health-technology-pandemic-prediction/
64. AI2 and Microsoft join the White House's push to enlist AI for the war on coronavirus https://www.geekwire.com/2020/ai2-microsoft-team-tech-leaders-use-ai-war-coronavirus/
65. How AI Tracks the Coronavirus Spread https://www.usnews.com/news/best-countries/articles/2020-03-11/how-scientists-are-using-artificial-intelligence-to-track-the-coronavirus

Chapter 2
AI-Enabled Technologies that Fight the Coronavirus Outbreak

Development of innovative designs, new applications, new technologies and heavier investment in AI are continued to be seen every day. However, with the sudden impact of COVID19, so severe and urgent around the world, adoption of AI is propelled to an unprecedent level, because it helps to fight the virus pandemic by enabling one or more of the following possibilities: (1) autonomous everything, (2) pervasive knowledge, (3) assistive technology and (4) rational decision support. The deployment of AI into these aspects may be bold and experimental, but it is in full force, all scales, unanimous and swift in timing which may otherwise take years. The four aspects which are enabled by AI changed our lifestyle, so did the coronavirus. It is almost like a revolution in speeding up the technologies and their adoption in a short time. The following showcases a series of examples of technologies which are infused with AI for provision of one or more of the four benefits, with the aim of fighting the coronavirus and of course saving lives. In particular, the examples show how AI as a technological enabler enhances the existing process for fulfilling one or more of the four benefits.

2.1 Infection Risk Identification

As the first line of defence against COVID-19 pandemic, in-home risk assessment is a protocol by which anybody can check for himself or somebody else at home whether he/she has contracted the coronavirus through some basic tests. The assessment involves a dialogue of questions to which the subject has to answer using a questionnaire based on how he feels and where he has visited. The responses of the questionnaire are taken to some medical experts for analysis, deciding the infection risk level of that person. Using ICT and AI, however, this assessment can be fully digitized.

S. J. Fong et al., *Artificial Intelligence for Coronavirus Outbreak*,
SpringerBriefs in Computational Intelligence,
https://doi.org/10.1007/978-981-15-5936-5_2

A mobile app is being developed by the Laboratory for Theory and Mathematical Modelling in the Division of Infectious Diseases at Augusta University [1] that allows users to DIY the risk assessment at home. AI is applied for replacing the human expert judgement on deciding the risk level based on the answers received from the mobile app. The app queries the user-related information to possible infection of coronavirus, such as common symptoms (fever, headache, dry cough, breathing difficulty and fatigue) and their duration and severity, travel history, work and residential information and demographics. Some sample screenshots of such mobile app are shown in Fig. 2.1 as an example.

The information will be processed by AI algorithm which computes the risk level and classifies the user to be one of the following groups: high risk, moderate risk, low risk, no risk, etc. Although it is unknown exactly which AI algorithm was used in any particular mobile app which probably is a commercial secret especially for non-government organizations, the logic behind is usually a set of decision rules. These decision rules will take a similar form as those presented in Fig. 2.2. The decision rules can be predefined by the developer while they could be updateable by

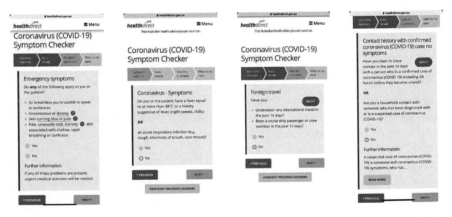

Fig. 2.1 Illustration of mobile app which checks the well-being of the user for identifying infection

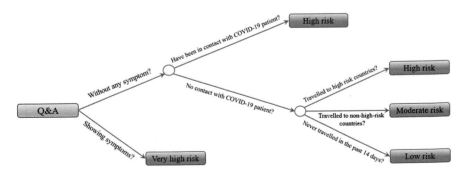

Fig. 2.2 Example of decision rules that are generated by AI algorithm

the vendor, or learnt over time by AI, or a hybrid of expert tuning and automated machine learning. In machine learning, which is one of the main disciplinaries of AI, this is typical task of classification by supervised learning, where some historical samples are used to induce a representative model which remembers the mapping between the attributes and the prediction classes. The supervised learning algorithms [2] for building a classification model range from simple Bayesian network, Decision tree, Support vector machine to sophisticated neural network and deep learning, just to name a few. Once the decision rules are induced from the classification model, they are ready to divert a new set of survey sample which is inputted into the app, to one of the specific class. A series of conditional tests are performed at the intermediate nodes in the decision rules, over the input survey data. An outcome is generated at the end of the decision rules, which would feedback to the user via the app.

Further from individually classifying users into risk groups based on their submitted information, AI plays a role in something bigger at the back-end server. The information collected from many users will be pooled together for piecing into a full picture of the regional virus outbreak using big data analytics. Some useful insights such as the epicentres, how the virus circulated, propagated and the risk levels in each suburb, can be known through this collective information from many users. Clusters of hot groups could be identified over the densities of infested cases, from. Technically, collecting this information and analysing it are possible, assuming privacy concerns are taken care of (anonymizing the data). There are three challenges that need to be conquered here: (1) AI smart algorithms which automatically identify the past and current high-risk areas and possibly predict the future nearby regions; at the same time, the risk levels and the propagation rate would also be computed. (2) the cloud processing and big data infrastructure that are required to support thousands of users' information submission and requests for the latest collective updated results. (3) visualization for large-scale geographical data.

In this scenario, AI algorithms related to spatial–temporal modelling [3] would be useful because the epidemic indeed spreads and travels in time, from town to town and city to city. The risk assessment data collected from a population of users are prefect ingredients feeding big data analytics which may embrace spatial–temporal modelling and prediction. In particular, a classical measure called Moran's I index [4] which computes spatial autocorrelation by simultaneously considering both feature values and their locations has been popularly used for predicting the risk levels of the next areas. Moran's I index is named after an Australian statistician, Emeritus Professor Patrick Alfred Pierce Moran. Moran found that spatial autocorrelation can be modelled by a complex spatial correlation among close proximity in space, which can be extended beyond 1-, 2-, 3-dimension and to however large multi-dimensional and multi-directional space. The Moran's I index for spatial autocorrelation is given as

$$Moran I = \frac{n}{S_0} \times \frac{\sum_{i=1}^{n} \sum_{j=1}^{n} w_{i,j} \times z_i \times z_j}{\sum_{i=1}^{n} z_i^2}, \tag{2.1}$$

where z_i is the deviation of an attribute for feature i from its mean $(x_i—X)$, $w_{i,j}$ is the spatial weight between feature i and j, which is the number of confirmed cases in $[i,j]$ coordinates of a 2D space, n is equal to the total number of features (confirmed cases) and S is the aggregate of all the spatial weights:

$$S_0 = \sum_{i=1}^{n} \sum_{j=1}^{n} w_{i,j} \tag{2.2}$$

The z_i-score for the statistic is computed as

$$z_I = \frac{I - E[I]}{\sqrt{V[I]}}, \tag{2.3}$$

where

$$E[I] = \frac{-1}{(n-1)} \tag{2.4}$$

$$V[I] = E[I^2] - E[I]^2. \tag{2.5}$$

The 3D concept of Moran's I theory has been widely used for modelling the autocorrelation of feature values (which could be interpreted as number of confirmed cases) across a two-dimensional space or map, plus the time dimension. Figure 2.3 shows an example of 3D concept in Moran's I index where the features in terms of number of confirmed cases, depicted in different colours are projected in time as heights of the columns on a 2D map.

In the literature, there have been many prediction models formulated which are based on Moran's I theory for predicting the spread of virus outbreak. Moran's

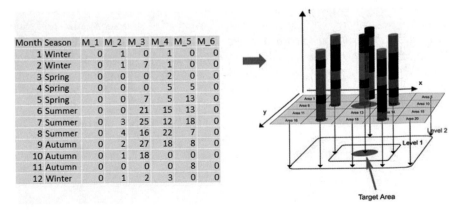

Month	Season	M_1	M_2	M_3	M_4	M_5	M_6
1	Winter	0	1	0	1	0	0
2	Winter	0	1	7	1	0	0
3	Spring	0	0	0	2	0	0
4	Spring	0	0	0	5	5	0
5	Spring	0	0	7	5	13	0
6	Summer	0	0	21	15	13	0
7	Summer	0	3	25	12	18	0
8	Summer	0	4	16	22	7	0
9	Autumn	0	2	27	18	8	0
10	Autumn	0	1	18	0	0	0
11	Autumn	0	0	0	0	8	0
12	Winter	0	1	2	3	0	0

Fig. 2.3 Illustration of how the seasonality of virus outbreaks is incorporated into the spatial–temporal computation model [5]

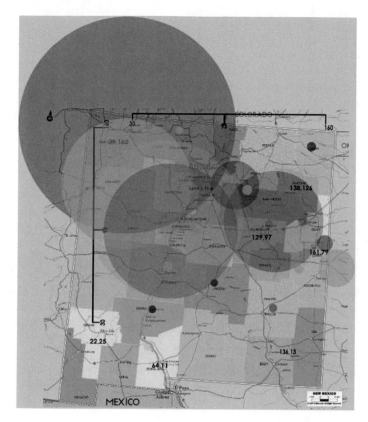

Fig. 2.4 Clusters of predicted next outbreak locations with the size of cluster representing the severity

I index is often used in conjunction of AI algorithms, such as clustering which allows similar data objects to merge into segments or clusters automatically and time-series forecasting which projects future values by modelling the current trend. Figure 2.4 shows the risk levels of nearby regions as an example illustrating the potential neighbouring areas from the epicentre can be computed by Moran's I index and clustering algorithm. Readers are referred to [5] for more details.

2.2 Smart Screening for High Body Temperature

Mobile app with AI that assesses the risk level of users at home or anywhere else is a thin line of defence relying on the honesty of the users who answer the questions truthfully. In some busy public places, like airports, train stations, office buildings, schools and hospitals, mass screening in an effort of detecting visitors who carry symptoms of COVID-19 disease is necessary. High body temperature is one of the most common symptoms in COVID-19. Decades ago, traditional thermal scanning technology checked users one by one, moving sequentially in a queue and stopping by in front of the camera for a second or so, for accurate detection. Recent Infrared Thermal Image Scanners (ITIS) technology has been widely deployed at border controls for the mass screening of travellers for fever symptoms. ITIS was put under test by a team of researchers from University of Otago, Dunedin, New Zealand, for measuring their front-of-face performance at airports. It was found that ITIS in detecting fever performed moderately well, with the area under Receiver Operating Characteristic (ROC) curves at 0.86 which is approximately at accuracy level of 95% with confidence intervals 0.75–0.97 [6].

A new generation of screening is needed for speeding up the mass screening process and improving the accuracy in fever detection. The state-of-the-art ITIS technologies often are equipped with AI functions which automatically pinpoint each human face from a crowd and focus on just the right facial point for measuring the body temperature. This not only saves time by filtering out the unwanted regions of the whole image, but also can focus and better analyse those small areas of interest. Therefore, the accuracy could be improved, and false alarm rate is reduced with the appropriate optical equipment and the AI functions. For example, a cup of hot coffee that is being held in a traveller's hand will be excluded in the body temperature measurement. By this way, the screening system is able to handle mass detection over a crowd of walking travellers. Figure 2.5 shows a snapshot of thermal image captured by ITIS over multiple targets. Fast speed and strong processing power are needed should many people on the move are needed to be measured simultaneously.

In a nutshell, the core of this AI function is rapid detection and tracking in thermal infrared imagery, powered by computer vision algorithms. The algorithms are largely divided into two groups: detection and tracking, which first identifies the areas of interest (human faces) over a background and follows their movement until out of view for avoiding multi-triggered detection, respectively. Detecting body temperature on human face requires outlining the human body shape from the background and then finding the face area which is relatively the warmest surface because it is not covered by clothes. To this end, thresholding technique and extracting human body shape information from images [7, 8] would be useful. For enhancing accuracy

Fig. 2.5 A snapshot of thermal image by ITIS empowered by AI for multi-targets monitoring

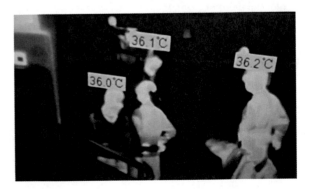

performance, some research works are geared towards a hybrid use of both thermal imagery and visual of the same scene [9].

On the other hand, tracking is about locating the trajectory of a moving person over time. One of the common ways is to start with an initial human face detection and then performs the same detection by recognition of nearby detection areas is repeated over time. The underlying AI algorithms are known as two broad categories—appearance-based methods and point-based methods. The former group of methods induces a model of the tracking object which allows continuous updates as it moves. It can be done based on the contour [10] called active contour [11] coupled with energy minimization function for shape matching or based on the template which is a frame outlined from the object at the initial detection. Template tracking is then a matter of matching regions of the scene that best match the frame and updating the template iteratively as the new appearance may gradually change in time [12]. For example, the displacement between the object and the fixed angle of the camera distorts the template away from the original template. In some probabilistic template-based tracking model, a prediction of where the next frame is most likely to be located based on the trajectory helps speed-up the search of the next matching frame [13].

The other groups of methods, namely, point-based methods are using pixels or points in a scene which represents the current coordinate of the moving object with reference to the coordinates of other objects in a scene. In this case of multi-target tracking, several popular image filters can be used, ranging from the simplest to the sophisticated, such as Linear Kalman filter, Global Nearest Neighbour filter and Joint Probabilistic Data Association filter, just to name a few. The concept is to associate each detection in each temporal frame (which are generated at high speed for high-resolution thermal and/or visual camera) to a trajectory, while the trajectory is monitored and remember along the way. Readers are referred to [14] for more information about multi-target tracking along with detecting anomalies in body temperature by ITIS. In general, multi-target detection and tracking is a broad topic. Many research endeavours have been committed to this topic which can be categorized according to a taxonomy as shown in Fig. 2.6. The research is still ongoing worldwide, with the prime objective of increasing the screening accuracy, coverage and speed.

2.3 Deep Learning and Radiological Image Analysis

Checking body temperature and risk assessment by questionnaire are the only entry level in COVID-19 diagnosis. By far the most common diagnostic pathway for COVID-19 currently is collecting and analysing RNA specimen of body fluid collected from the testee. The principle is to observe the outcome of adding a special enzyme called 'Reverse Transcriptase' (RT-PCA) to the RNA specimen, producing a two-stranded DNA. Under fluorescent dye, a tester can tell whether the test turns positive for COVID-19 when the DNA multiply upon adding the nucleotides. If no multiplication of the DNA is observed, the testee is free from COVID-19 infection.

Fig. 2.6 Taxonomy of multi-targets detection and tracking for mass thermal screening

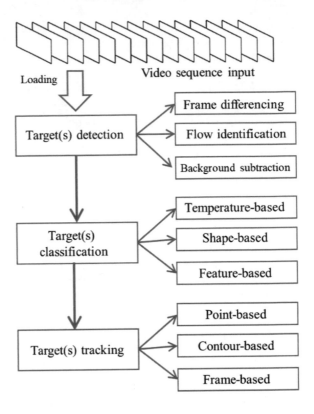

Based on this RT-PCA principle, quick paper-kit test within half an hour is made possible for the frontline healthcare staff. The paper-kit is a mini incubator for the observation of fusing the viral proteins of a sputum specimen to the antibodies. However, the accuracy level of such paper test-kit could be as low as 60% while false alarm rate remains high [15].

An alternative method for COVID-19 test is medical imaging-based diagnosis, which is more accurate in general but requires expensive equipment operated by radiologists. A Computerized Tomography (CT) scan of a patient's chest which is a series of X-ray images from cross sections of the lung at different depths. Should the patient be infected with COVID-19, the CT scan of the lung reveals tissues of irregularity. The anomalies are subtle and hard to be distinguished between that of COVID-19 and that of viral pneumonia. The characteristics of COVID-19 as appeared on CT scan include but not limited to air space contraction, murky paving shades, peripheral ground glass opacities, traction bronchiectasis and bronchovesicular thickening [15]. Overall, CT-based COVID-19 diagnosis is found to be better than RT-PCR test, having sensitivity measure between 80 and 90% [16].

AI is an epitome of how leading-edge technology can help analyse CT scans of COVID-19 patients. It is accepted worldwide that AI is a good assistant along with CT assessment, not only for COVID-19 but in many cancers related diagnosis.

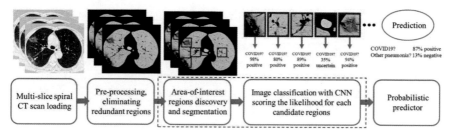

Fig. 2.7 Computer-aided COVID-19 diagnosis from CT scan

Subsequently, prototypes of AI algorithms especially deep learning which has excellent ability of non-linear modelling have been built by a number of research teams for aiding COVID-19 detection on chest CT scans. Research lab funded by Alibaba claims that their AI-based image recognition tool yields an accuracy level of 96% in distinguishing pneumonia caused COVID-19 from that of other causes [17]. A latest medical report, by Gozes, O. et al., claims that their new thoracic AI algorithm powered by deep learning over CT scans is reaching 98.2% sensitivity and 92.2% specificity, it is fast as well [18].

How exactly AI in the name of deep learning help improve the CT scan diagnosis for COVID-19 patients? AI may neither be replacing the radiologist when it comes to operating a professional CT scanning nor taking over the final decision in confirming the diagnosis verdict. However, AI has been applied for decades as a supplementary decision support tool, used by radiologist for doing fast analysis, in addition to experts' visual inspection. The AI diagnosis module usually inputs a set of CT scans manually or semi-automatically by wiring the workstation that connects to the imaging peripheral. Often the output is a diagnosis report indicating the likelihood of each possible outcome, based on the computed results through the AI algorithm. The diagnosis report would be used as a reference for the doctors to make a final decision. This is how the AI computerized process works, as shown in Fig. 2.7. Firstly, the multi-sliced spiral set of CT scans is loading into a computer where AI is installed. The raw images would be pre-processed, mainly by subtracting the background, correcting the orientation of the images and placing the lung cross-sectional image from each scan in a prominent position showing the lesions and organs. Other data transformation may apply, as some researchers prefer to apply some image/signal processing filters for improving the clarity of the image. In the second step, data segmentation algorithm apply here for identifying and distinguishing the areas of interest from the lung image. Extracting the so-called salient features is one of the most important parts of the process; the efficacy of machine learning hence the accuracy of the final output, depends very much on the good quality image feeds prior to the neural network. In the earlier days, image segmentation was a separate process requiring edge detection and data clustering methods. Areas of interest were manually highlighted over the CT scan images, cropping the shapes and their textures within, then feeding them into machine learning model for recognition and classification. Since millennia, deep learning has become a promising approach for its image processing capability to effectively mark out and segment the areas of interest from the CT scans. Each area of interest would be evaluated for the likelihood of belonging to a COVID-19 class or something else. A final merger collectively decides based on the likelihood of each region whether the patient is suffering from COVID-19 disease or other pneumonia. This could be implemented by some probabilistic reasoning tools such as Bayesian network which generates a final outcome with probability associated. All the possible outcomes and their probabilities serve as good reference for doctors to make final conclusions in a timely manner.

How does deep learning help in the process as in Fig. 2.7? There have been many hypes and praises on the efficacy of deep learning, tautologically known as Convolution Neural Network (CNN). CNN is one of the latest variants of neural network inheriting the basic neural structure, like neurons and their connectivity among intermediate layers, learnable weights associated with each link, activation function and bias. A neuron receives an input value from its preceding links, multiplies these values with their weights, applies an activation function over the weighted values and responds with a new value which in turn passes on to its subsequent layer of neurons. The number of neurons required at the input layer is equal to the number of pixels on a CT scan which typically is in DICOM format. DICOM is abbreviation for Digital Imaging and Communications in Medicine, commonly for archiving and transferring high-resolution medical images among Picture Archiving And Communication Systems (PACS). Behind the input layer of neurons, there are several intermediate layers of neurons called feature maps. The feature maps also are commonly known as convolutional layers because they convolve the outputs from the input layers via some filters. The purpose of convolution is to extract important features; the convolution proceeds through several layers of feature maps, filtering out the unimportant and retaining the important features out in each layer. The feature maps collectively are known as kernels; their size is to be arbitrarily chosen by the designer. As shown in Fig. 2.8, subsampling and convolution happen across the kernels, condensing the whole CT scan image to specific areas of interest from the input layer to the latter layer. This is done by the efforts of each neuron responding at each feature map to an interesting area of the previous feature map. How does it define interestingness? It depends on the types and number of convolutional filters chosen, usually the filters are magnifying up the salient features over a large area

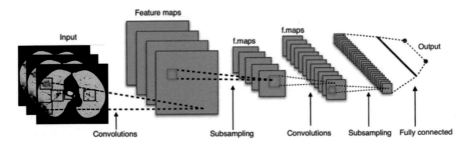

Fig. 2.8 A typical CNN structure for COVID-19 diagnosis from CT scan

and suppressing down the major and ordinary areas. After a feature map is 'convoluted and sub-sampled', the selected output has become concise which is known as activation map where the effect of applying the filter has been highlighted. Between the activation maps, there is some activation function controlling how much or how little convolution should happen in a non-linear fashion, based on the weights at the links between neurons across successive feature maps. Near the output there is some pooling layer which is designed to consolidate the dimensionality of the activation's map out, preventing the dimensionality becomes too large. This could be done optionally by either max-pooling or average-pooling strategy. At the end, high-level abstractions can be achieved from the fully connected set of kernels (feature maps) and pooling layers. The key features are the essential details that characterize each area of interest which are quality ingredients for supervised learning. Then the whole CNN can continue to run until it reaches some equilibrium. The whole process is iterative similar to the learning cycles by backpropagation neural network. The weights at the neuron links are continuously updated while training samples are fed, until a stage when no longer error reduction can be observed or the discriminant between two successive cycle falls below a predefined threshold. Readers are referred to [19] for more information as there are many variants of CNN; almost a new or modified model is proposed and published by academic journals every week.

Since January 2019, medical staff at radiology department of Zhongnan Hospital, China started using AI software to screen typical or partial visual signs of lung pneumonia manifested by COVID-19 from CT scans. The speed and convenience gained by the AI software relieve frontline healthcare workers as well as hospital radiologists from their overloaded duties. The speed-up of the process helps not only in diagnosis, but the efficiency extends to deciding who to isolate, who are confirmed, what treatments should be appropriate, etc. Even the slightest speed-up means a lot in saving lives as the hospitals in Wuhan were quickly overwhelmed by increasingly large number of patients like tsunami in a very short time, as the virus hit hard in Wuhan in January and February. The AI software alone, however, does not confirm whether a person has contracted the disease or not, but it offers good indication with reasonable accuracy on recognizing a pneumonia condition from the lung images of CT scans. The indication is useful for diagnosis that would have to be followed up with other lab tests and further observations. InferVision is one of the pioneer developers of AI-based COVID-19 diagnosis software, whose product was intensively used by 34 hospitals in China, examined lung images of CT scans from over 32,000 suspected cases. The processing time was reported to have reduced from typically 15 min to 3 min. InferVision which is a Beijing company backed by Google Sequoia Capital is an example of how AI software was deployed in such large scale at the soonest possible timing since the early days of outbreak. A screenshot of the AI-based COVID-19 software is shown in Fig. 2.9. It can be seen that the GUI is carefully design with a futuristic calming blue and black theme which causes minimum distraction; the output of the AI diagnosis is abstract and stands out in the center, conveying critical information to the users at an easy glance. Secondary information and details are at the sides. Allowing medical staff at the crucial time to stay focused, calm and be well informed by AI diagnosis is very important. On

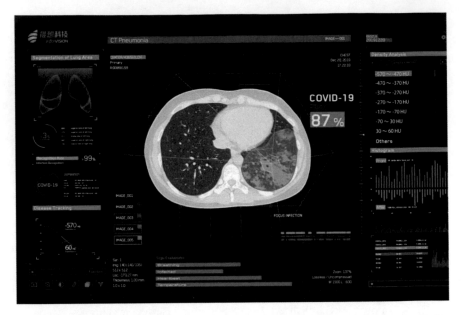

Fig. 2.9 The GUI of an AI software for COVID-19 diagnosis (image courtesy by Beijing InferVision Technology Co., Ltd.)

11 March 2020, it is reported that InferVision AI diagnosis software was exported to Japan, as a global effort to help medical staff doing screening and to stop virus spreading as early as possible.

This is also another example of technology adoption at critical time, where it may not be ideal to have developed and tested an AI software in such a short time. But the mourning of victims suffered from COVID-19 and snowballing death tolls indeed forced researchers and developers to push ahead of what the best efforts that they could do on hand, even as a contingency plan but with great urgency. It is believed that future works on further enhancing the AI algorithms are ongoing, in terms of speed and accuracy. Other aspects of enhancement on Infervision's GUI would be NLP and remote gesture recognition which could further speed-up the human and computer interaction time.

2.4 AI-Driven Unmanned Technologies

AI has so far helped health risk assessment, detection of potential patients at gantries and fast radiological diagnosis in hospitals, in the form of AI software running at a workstation or smartphone, separating the sick from the healthy people. At this time of crisis, how possible is it that AI will be augmenting or even replacing healthcare workers or caregivers for the sake of reducing the human contacts? As a safety measure of social distancing, the less intensity of human touch means lower infection risk for the human workers. This time of COVID-19 spells out a sad irony—nobody community nor government alone can fight this invisible enemy of the century, but borders are sealed and physical teamwork is impossible; healthcare workers know the best about the importance of social distancing, but their duties put them at great risk by working most closely with the patients and the suspected; elders need most interactions and emotional supports during this gloomy pandemic, but they are the priority group to be strictly isolated because they are the vulnerable to the virus; and police officers should be patrolling against looting and burglary, but they are tasked to chase every civilian to stay at home. All these mentioned tasks have one thing in common which must be either eliminated or minimized at all costs—reduction of human interaction. One apparent solution is robotics, which has a long history in providing human with automation and abilities of performing tasks in all walks of life, varying from ATM machines, supermarket kiosks to sophisticated surgical assistance on operating tables. In this section, the applications of robotics that are powered by AI at hospital, home and public places are explored.

2.4.1   Robotics with AI at Hospital

Hospitals can be hotspots of contagion due to frequent visits of patients confirmed or suspected. Regular sanitization is of upmost importance to ensure the safety of workers, patients and visitors. Robots are the best candidates for this risky job because they are machines and naturally impossible for virus infection. Similar to floor-cleaning bots which have been commercially available as consumers products, autonomous robots can do more than cleaning in hospitals. There have been robots deployed during the COVID-19 pandemic in hospital for doing the following tasks where humans are suspectable to contagion (Fig. 2.10).

Fig. 2.10 Mobile UV lampworking in action killing germs in hospital

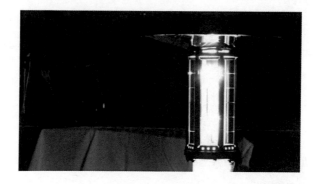

(1) Robots that are equipped with germicidal lamps able to roam around indoor while disinfecting surfaces with specific types of UV light—UV-C radiation which is also known as Ultraviolet Germicidal Irradiation (UVGI). UV-C/UVGI has been commonly used in waste treatment plants and laboratories for hospital grade of strong disinfection. The unique features which are enabled by AI include self-navigation, computer vision, optimization of shortest-path, maximum cleaning areas, object avoidance, etc.

(2) Caregiver robots that mimic behaviours of nurses and health workers in performing basic housekeeping operations. For example, food and drug deliveries, waste collection, measuring patients' vital signals, serving meals, etc. A humanoid serving robot called Amigo prototyped by RoboEarth which is a European-funded project is developed with collaboration of five European universities. Amigo is able to perform simple task to patient like handing over a glass of drink with its pincer hand and aware of the objects and patient around him. Far from being able to accomplish sophisticated tasks like a human nurse interacting with patients, robots are not affected by fatigues due to heavy workload and more importantly virus infection, making it a perfect machine for field work of contagion and for long hours between battery charging. Due to the emergency of the COVID-19 outbreak and sky-rocketing death toll, Spanish authorities committed to purchasing four robots that are able to automate testing processes with the suspected patients. The robots which are designed to perform COVID-19 tests and simple vital monitoring tasks, without sophisticated abilities to do complex interactions with the patients, can increase the COVID-19 tests from 20,000 a day to 80,000 with the aid of AI algorithms. The four robots indeed help reduce the risk of exposing human healthcare workers at the frontline to the virus. The AI functions would include those mentioned above, plus localization, fine-tuning of motor movements (e.g. picking up a glass and handing it gently to a patient) and perhaps specialized motor skills pertaining to COVID-19 tests such as throat swab in cooperation with computer vision (Fig. 2.11).

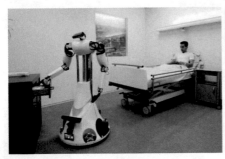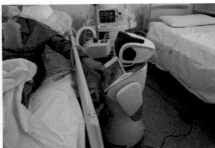

Fig. 2.11 Patient-care robots: Amigo robot in the lab at Eindhoven Technical University (image courtesy of Bart van Overbeeke/Tech United Eindhoven). A robot providing interactive dialogues and information with ICU patients in an Italian hospital (image courtesy of Associate Press)

(3) A blood sampling robot called Automated Venipuncture Device (AVD) in response to the overwhelming workload of medical staff especially nurses in hospitals since the outbreak of coronavirus was created, by a joint research team of Rutgers University and Robert Wood Johnson University Hospital. The new device can automatically locate the best location of an insertion point on a blood vein and draws blood sample quickly and accurately—on par or better than a human can do. It is known that drawing blood from obviously visible veins called palpable veins is relatively with just one shot even by rookie nurses. Failing the first attempt means the need of second needle insertion or more, adding extra pain to the patients and consuming precious time for the nurses. During the COVID-19 crisis, AVD is called to the frontline, aiding nurses to take blood samples efficiently. The efficiency is reported from experimental results that were published in [20]. Success rate of 87% was achieved over 31 testing volunteers, in comparison to manual insertion by human at success rate between 27% and 60%. Human has a relatively large variation for it depends on the experience of the nurse, the difficulty of access to the veins, lighting, conditions of the skins and muscles, etc.

However, AVD is still a machine prototype though it has been catalyzed to speed-up by the pandemic for relieving the workloads of the medical personnel. There is still room for improvement of the accuracy rate especially for cases involved difficult-to-access veins and unstable environment, for example, ambulance ride or airborne hospital transport. The underlying technologies for AVD are threefold. Firstly, it needs a robotic arm with a precision engineered system of motors which positions and inserts a needle at the right spot, right force and right time on the arm. Secondly, the placement of the needle is guided by a combined signals of Near-Infrared (NIR) light and ultrasound imaging, and AI algorithm which chooses one of the most suitable veins and the best part of the vein for cannulation. The choice of location is selected by algorithm based on the 3D reconstructs of the imaging signals from both NIR and ultrasound. And the depth of insertion is carefully calculated from the 3D images, so once the needle pierces through the skin it can accurately and swiftly penetrate right into the centre of the vein lumen. Thirdly, the AVD is an integrated system that combines the imaging and AI functions mentioned above. It has a built-in refrigerated sample storage and centrifuge which analyses blood samples and generating reports on the spot (Fig. 2.12).

(4) Robots at the hospital triage—Cruzr is a model of service robot developed by a Chinese company UBTECH and deployed in use during COVID-19 epidemic in People's Hospital of Shenzhen. It is designed for high efficiency, for example, real-time tracking of 200 patients' body temperature per minute; nurses would be notified immediately should anybody be detected feverish. Cruzr and its team are now working in Royal Brisbane and Women's Hospital and Princess Alexandra Hospital as service assistant at triage, directing patients to different sections. The robots are equipped with AI for working autonomously and independently, connected to 5G cloud network as a team in hospital. Human control is totally spared without the need to control or command the robots. A new batch of

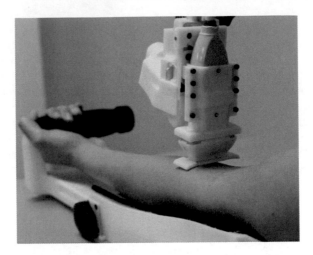

Fig. 2.12 AVD prototype that draws and analyses blood with a built-in centrifuge (image courtesy of Rutgers)

Cruzr will be working at hospital in Melbourne in April 2020. They are part of the medical crew without getting tired or infected during COVID-19. When they were working in Shenzhen back to January and February this year, they were dispatched to spray disinfectants inside and around the hospital areas in self-driving mode (Fig. 2.13).

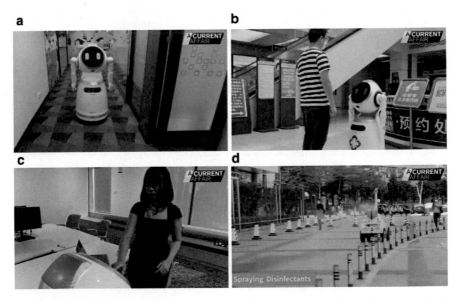

Fig. 2.13 Cruzr working in action—**a** patrolling, **b** serving patients at triage, **c** information kiosk, and **d** spraying disinfectant. (image courtesy of Current Affair)

2.4.2 Robotics with AI at Home

Fear arose as the epidemic first emerged, causing much panic and changing everybody's lifestyle at the time of crisis. The outbreak of COVID-19 has grown into a global pandemic killing hundred of thousands lives. Governments of many countries ordered for social distancing and stay-home lockdown curfew as a means to slow down the virus spread. At the same time, fear of death is instilled in everybody's mind. News of mass infection and death suddenly have overwhelmed us from almost every country around the world. In this darkest period, from bad to worse, we were told to stay home, isolated, and cut off physical contacts from our social circles. This psychological trauma has impacted us a lot, especially the elders group who are most vulnerable to the virus. Under self-isolation, the elders may suffer from loneliness, fear and depression (Fig. 2.14).

Research team from Heriot-Watt University, led by Professor Oliver Lemon, dedicated to design a pioneer robot for accompanying elders at home, which is particularly useful during the outbreak of coronavirus. The main feature of the robot is its provision of conversational AI human–robot interaction. Put simply, it is a speech interface built into a machine which can converse with the elders naturally like how a human do. A specific name for this type of robots is Socially Assistive Robots (SARS) which is capable of caregiving and performing simple tasks in addition to conversing with elders. SARS indeed relieve loneliness and stress, therefore, improving psychological well-being to the elders with 24/7 companionship. The techniques under the hood of SARS are an integration of computer vision, human–robot interaction which can be optimized by machine learning algorithms, localization, human activity recognition and analysis—through which SARS robot can know what the elder is doing, detecting whether he/she is in danger and figuring out what assistance he/she may need. To make the robot more human-like; for speech, Natural Language Processing (NLP) is applied; and for empathy, a new branch of AI called Emotional Intelligence (EI)

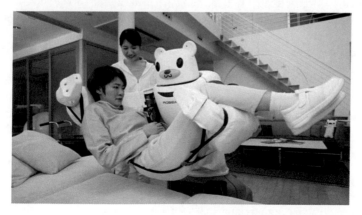

Fig. 2.14 Robear—a robot bear which is designed as both an assistive machine and NLP chatbot by a Japanese company Riken

has been exploited. Emotional intelligence is the capability to understand the elder's emotions from facial recognition, know about the responding emotions by sensing the elder's tune and words he/she used in the dialogue, and understand the effect of a conversation made with the elder. Amazon Alexa, a leading commercial company in NLP mobile App, released a conversational AI-based social robot, namely, Alana. A Beijing-based company called Turning specialized in designing chatbots which is a collection of NLP software programmes that can be embedded into any shell of humanoid or robot, giving it the ability to naturally and interactively chatting with elderly.

2.4.3 Robotics with AI at Public Places

Flying drones, Unmanned Aerial Vehicles (UAV) are being used during the pandemic to partially replace human activities in air, yet trying to meet or fulfil the need of societal activities. As a general rule of thumb, any human even law enforcer is put at risk of exposure to virus, when he has to do his field duty outdoor. Although nobody is allowed to roam on the street, certain orders and operations must still take place—these activities include but not limited to patrolling for detecting anybody who violates the social distancing rules, delivering foods and essential items, providing virtual tours of places of interest in lieu of human visits, and even walking your dogs on your behalf. All these activities if they had to be undertaken by merely mechanical flying drones, certain AI must be added to it, so to breathe life into those machines making them intelligent. The following is a list of examples where UAV is tasked to serve homebound residents during COVID-19.

Lockdown patrol—under the lockdown decree—pockets of people still irresponsibly roam at the streets ignoring the law and neglecting their infection risk. Authorities deploy squads of policemen to patrol around the public places, warning or fining them penalty. More effectively than human patrol, aerial surveillance using UAV through a bird eye view detects any human presence in the streets that are supposed to be empty. Patrol drones are not something totally new. The fundamental functions of UAV's which enable them to fly by specific scheduled routes are upgraded with extra useful functions for COVID-19. For instance, the UAV would need to tell whether the detected human is singular, in pair, trio or a gang; whether the person is wearing mask or not, whether the person is showing signs of illness, etc. and whether those people are getting too close to each other for social distancing. All these new functions specifically for COVID-19 need to be programmed by AI algorithms. The Chinese government was the pioneer in using UAVs coupled with thermal cameras to check out walking pedestrians who are sick from the sky. This technique was proven successful in scanning crowds to pick out COVID-19 carriers. Variants of such surveillance drones have emerged which have add-on capabilities of two-way audio—it can listen to sounds and allows a law enforcer to speak through the drone to the target people remotely. Other add-ons are navigation by lidar, object recognition, human activity recognition, video analytics, autonomous flying abilities, obstacle avoidance, etc. Although AI was the centrepiece of the UAV applications, human is still needed in some scenarios. For instance, AI and computer vision detail that there are crowds congregating and violating the social distancing rule; a human operator may need to yell through the loudspeaker to verbally persuade the crowd to disperse. The tone and the skills of negotiation, sometimes a sense of humour, are still done better by human. British police also adopted using UAV for chasing off crowds in the streets during COVID-19. But they took it a little further by taking photos of the violators and shame them on Tweeter, tweeting out their faces and times and places of violation for public display (Fig. 2.15).

Other than enforcing social distancing, some UAVs nick-named 'Tour Drones' are tasked for benevolent purposes with unique video recording and broadcasting functions and wide connectivity. Tour drones fly around well-known city centres, attractions, major transport hubs where used to be frequent by travellers. The drones with high-resolution video capture eerie scenes and real-time broadcast to viewers who are isolated at home. This serves as a good cabin fever remedy to anybody who is suffering from claustrophobic distress. The open view of quiet places including those which were used to be crowded or over-crowded provides a serene sensation

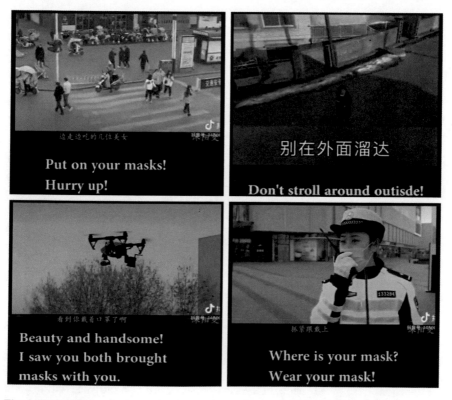

Fig. 2.15 UAV was warning pedestrians as law enforcement to wear masks in Beijing during COVID-19 lockdown

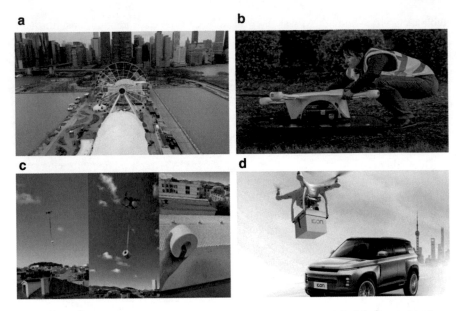

Fig. 2.16 UAVs are used for benevolent purposes during COVID-19 lockdown; **a** virtual tour of deserted streets in Chicago; **b** delivering medical samples; **c** delivering toilet paper in time of urgency and **d** delivering car keys in car rental business

that soothes restlessness and irritability. DJDrones is one of the pioneers in providing free footages of virtual tours over quarantined cities that could be watched online by anybody. Other benevolent and practical applications of UAV during COVID-19 are delivery of food, medicine and essential supplies, even toilet paper! (Fig. 2.16).

2.4.4 AI Beneath the Surface of Robots

Unmanned technologies have a long history since its inception to be powered by AI. The intelligent controls by AI transformed the mechanical automation largely to autonomous machines which embrace all the advantages of machinery (24/7, precision, and free from biohazard etc.). AI has added extra dimension of delicate functions. They are the 'intelligence' that comes from local knowledge from online analytics and sensing ability at the working environment, and global knowledge which offers deep insights from a macro-view by processing a massive amount of so-called big data. COVID-19 just served as a catalyst along the timeline of fusing AI into robotics, accelerating the pace of using the best of both at the time of crisis as a solace. It is anticipated that heavy investment and funding will continue to enhance the functionalities of AI robots in the near future. Current prototypes will become better, latest prototypes will mature, and new hybrid use of AI functions on robots would be attempted and tested. As a review, Table 2.1 summarizes some prominent

Table 2.1 Prominent AI functions found across robotic operations during COVID-19 lockdown

Applications	Extra AI techniques	Purposes
Sanitizing robots	Target identification by specific object recognition [27]; Optimization between coverage and intensity [28]	To guide the movement of the robot, for covering the areas for maximum disinfection. Along the way, the robot will have to recognize objects ahead and avoid colliding them
Blood test robots	Computer vision for NIR and ultrasound imaging [28]; auto venepuncture algorithms [29]	To allow a robot (station) identify the blood veins quickly and insert the needle accurately for efficient blood draw
Hospital triage robots	NLP [30]	To converse with visitors, medical staff and patients, offering them information and directions
Caregiving robots	NLP [30]; Emotional intelligence [31]; Chatbot algorithms [32]; Fall detection [33]	To provide emotional supports through artificial empathy and chatters to patients. It also monitors the safety of the patients at all times
Lockdown patrol UAVs	Human activity recognition [34]; Face recognition [35]; Symptoms identification [36]; Flight path optimization [37]	To assist law enforcement and warning people during pandemic lockdown; the UAVs need to identify distinguish people who are breaking the rules (e.g. gathering, not wearing masks), as well as sick
Delivery UAVs	Flight path optimization [37] Payload delivery optimization [38]	To facilitate unmanned supply delivery via the most optimized route, and ensure the payload is dropped in a safe manner

AI functions and their references that would have been applied in AI robotics during the COVID-19 crisis. The robotics applications do share common AI functions them. Ground robots generally require AI algorithms in localization [21], path finding [22] and computer vision [23] for autonomous navigation [24]. Medical robots would have higher requirements in image processing [25] for precision. UAVs require the on-par navigation capabilities to those ground robots, but with additional advances, such as balancing in the midst of wind turbulence [26].

References

1. Becky Brickwood, The power of AI in providing rapid at-home assessments of the coronavirus, The Health Europa, 6th March 2020. https://www.healtheuropa.eu/the-power-of-ai-in-provid ing-rapid-at-home-assessments-of-the-coronavirus/98350. Accessed 14 April 2020

2. Suthaharan S (2016) supervised learning algorithms. In: Machine learning models and algorithms for big data classification. Integrated Series in Information Systems, vol 36. Springer, Boston, MA, pp 183–206
3. Tryfona N, Price R, Jensen CS (2003) Chapter 3: Conceptual models for spatio-temporal applications. In: Sellis TK et al (eds) Spatio-temporal databases. Lecture Notes in Computer Science, vol 2520. Springer, Berlin, Heidelberg, pp 79–116
4. Moran PAP (1950) Notes on continuous stochastic phenomena. Biometrika 37(1):17–23
5. Lao KK, Deb S, Thampi SM, Fong S (2014) A novel disease outbreak prediction model for compact spatial-temporal environments. In: Thampi S, Gelbukh A, Mukhopadhyay J (eds) Advances in signal processing and intelligent recognition systems. Advances in Intelligent Systems and Computing, vol 264. Springer, pp 439–450
6. Priest PC, Duncan AR, Jennings LC, Baker MG (2011) Thermal image scanning for influenza border screening: results of an airport screening study. PLoS ONE 6(1):e14490. https://doi.org/10.1371/journal.pone.0014490
7. Zin TT, Takahashi R, Hama H (2007) Robust person detection using far infrared camera for image fusion. In: Innovative computing, information and control, 2007. ICICIC'07. Second International Conference on, pages 310–310, Sept 2007. https://doi.org/10.1109/icicic.2007.501
8. Wong WK, Chew ZY, Loo CK, Lim WS (2010) An effective trespasser detection system using thermal camera. In Computer Research and Development, 2010 Second International Conference on, pp 702–706, May 2010. https://doi.org/10.1109/iccrd.2010.161
9. Hwang JP, Kim N, Choi Y, Kweon IS (2015) Multispectral pedestrian detection: benchmark dataset and baseline. In: Computer vision and pattern recognition (CVPR), IEEE conference on, 2015
10. Yang M, Kpalma K, Ronsin J (2008) A survey of shape feature extraction techniques. In: Yin P-Y (ed), Pattern recognition, pp 43–90. IN-TECH, November 2008. 38 p
11. Kass M, Witkin A, Terzopoulos D (1988) Snakes: active contour models. Int J Comput Vis 1(4):321–331. ISSN 1573-1405. https://doi.org/10.1007/bf00133570
12. Matthews TI, Baker S (2004) The template update problem. Pattern Anal Mach Intell IEEE Trans 26(6):810–815. ISSN 0162-8828. https://doi.org/10.1109/tpami.2004.16
13. Smeulders AWM, Chu DM, Cucchiara R, Calderara S, Dehghan A, Shah M (2014) Visual tracking: an experimental survey. Pattern Anal Mach Intell IEEE Trans 36(7):1442–1468. ISSN 0162-8828. https://doi.org/10.1109/tpami.2013.230
14. Blackman S, Popoli R (1999) Design and analysis of modern tracking systems. Artech House radar library. Artech House, Boston, London. ISBN 1-580-53006-0
15. Moore CM, Bell DJ, COVID-19. https://radiopaedia.org/articles/covid-19-2. Accessed 19 March 2020
16. Hou H et al (2019) Correlation of Chest CT and RT-PCR Testing in Coronavirus Disease 2019 (COVID-19) in China: A Report of 1014 Cases Tao. 2019
17. Kharpal A (20202) China's giants from Alibaba to Tencent ramp up health tech efforts to battle coronavirus. https://www.cnbc.com/2020/03/04/coronavirus-china-alibaba-tencent-baidu-boost-health-tech-efforts.html. Accessed 19 March 2020
18. Gozes O et al (2020) Rapid AI development cycle for the Coronavirus (COVID-19) Pandemic : Initial Results for Automated Detection & Patient Monitoring using Deep Learning CT Image Analysis Article Type : Authors: Summary Statement : Key Results : List of abbreviations : Submitt Radiol Artif Intell
19. Hesamian MH, Jia W, He X et al (2019) Deep learning techniques for medical image segmentation: achievements and challenges. J Digit Imaging 32:582–596. https://doi.org/10.1007/s10278-019-00227-x
20. Leipheimer JM, Balter ML, Chen AI, Pantin EJ, Davidovich AE, Labazzo KS, Yarmush ML (2019) First-in-human evaluation of a hand-held automated venipuncture device for rapid venous blood draws. Technology 7(3–4):98–107
21. Castellanos JA, Tardós JD (1999) Mobile robot localization and map building: A Multisensor fusion approach, Springer, XIII, 205 p

22. Koubaa A, Bennaceur H, Chaari I, Trigui S, Ammar A, Sriti M-F, Alajlan M, Cheikhrouhou O, Javed Y (2018) Robot path planning and cooperation: foundations, algorithms and experimentations, Springer, 190 p, ISBN 978-3-319-77042-0

23. Sergiyenko O, Flores-Fuentes W, Mercorelli P (Eds), Machine vision and navigation, 2020, Springer, ISBN 978-3-030-22587-2

24. Chatterjee A, Rakshit A, Nirmal Singh N (2013) Vision based autonomous robot navigation algorithms and implementations, Springer, ISBN 978-3-642-33965-3

25. Paulsen RR, Moeslund TB (2020) Introduction to medical image analysis, Springer, ISBN 978-3-030-39363-2

26. Duan K, Fong S, Zhuang Y, Song W (2018) Artificial neural networks in coordinated control of multiple hovercrafts with unmodeled terms. Appl Sci 8:862

27. Treiber MA (2010) An introduction to object recognition: selected algorithms for a wide variety of applications, Springer, ISBN 978-1-84996-235-3

28. Chen Alvin I, Balter Max L, Maguire Timothy J, Yarmush Martin L (2016) 3D near infrared and ultrasound imaging of peripheral blood vessels for real-time localization and needle guidance. Med Image Comput Comput Assist Interv 9902:388–396

29. Balter ML, Chen AI, Maguire TJ, Yarmush ML (1982) Adaptive kinematic control of a robotic venipuncture device based on stereo vision, ultrasound, and force guidance. IEEE Trans Ind Electron 64(2):1626–1635

30. Kamath U, Liu J, Whitaker J (2019) Deep learning for NLP and speech recognition, Springer, ISBN 978-3-030-14596-5

31. Ayanoglu H, Duarte E (2019) Emotional design in human-robot interaction: theory, methods and applications, Springer, Human–Computer Interaction Series, ISBN 978-3-319-96722-6

32. Følstad A, Araujo T, Papadopoulos S, Law EL-C, Granmo O-C, Luger E, Brandtzaeg PB (Eds), Chatbot research and design, Springer, ISBN 978-3-030-39540-7

33. Ren Lingmei, Peng Yanjun (2019) Research of fall detection and fall prevention technologies: a systematic review. Access IEEE 7:77702–77722

34. Yu Z, Wang Z (2020) Human behavior analysis: sensing and understanding, Springer, ISBN 978-981-15-2109-6

35. Berle I (2020) Face recognition technology, Springer, ISBN 978-3-030-36887-6

36. Güttler J, Georgoulas C, Bock T (2016) Contactless fever measurement based on thermal imagery analysis, 2016 IEEE sensors applications symposium (SAS), 30 May 2016

37. Zhao P, Yang Y, Zhang Y, Bian K, Song L, Qiao P, Li Z (2018) Optimal trajectory planning of Drones for 3D mobile sensing, IEEE, 2018 IEEE global communications conference (GLOBECOM), 9-13 Dec. 2018

38. Alshanbari R, Khan S, El-Atab N, Mustafa Hussain M (2020) AI powered unmanned aerial vehicle for payload transport application, 2019 IEEE national aerospace and electronics conference (NAECON), 09 April 2020

Chapter 3
AI-Empowered Data Analytics for Coronavirus Epidemic Monitoring and Control

Governments and authorities knew little about the virus since the emergency of COVID-19 outbreak. The Chinese government upon the discovery of the early patients in Wuhan, informed WHO on 31 December 2019, as pneumonia of unknown causes. Epidemiologists, data scientists and biostatisticians have been working hand-in-hand for a common mission of trying to characterize and understand the characteristics of the infection as well as the virus itself, which is SARS alike. In front of an unknown disease which is so contagious and dangerous, governments and organization of both private and public started an all out approach using latest data analytics and AI algorithms in the hope of knowing more about the virus, so that the disease spread and progression could possibly be predicted. Data analytics and prediction are equally important if not more than the deployment of AI techniques in confronting the virus and assisting the treatment (as those techniques discussed in previous chapter). COVID-19 is an invisible enemy of mankind in microscopic scale. We can only know about its traits and behaviours as a posteriori knowledge from the collected data and statistics like chasing shadow. This chapter introduces and discusses how some of the prominent AI and data analytics examples that crunch over the data during COVID-19, for forecast and insights.

3.1 AI Predicted COVID-19 Outbreak Before It Happened

Was COVID-19 predicted accurately or by chance by AI prior to its arrival? A Canadian company called BlueDot [1] might have an answer, claiming that they had picked up signals and warned the official about the new disease ahead of WHO and CDC. The prediction was said to have come from scientific inference from an AI model by constantly monitoring the changes from various information sources in lieu of watching over the official statistics of daily reported cases.

S. J. Fong et al., *Artificial Intelligence for Coronavirus Outbreak*,
SpringerBriefs in Computational Intelligence,
https://doi.org/10.1007/978-981-15-5936-5_3

The AI algorithm which of course was kept commercially confidential builds an adaptive model which represents the potential of disease outbreak considering over multiple sources of salient information that are relevant to the disease development. These information sources contain tell-tale-signs hidden in massive amount of data, which could be filtered and discovered by data mining techniques. The tell-tale-signs could be but not limited to the following activities, which can be technically obtained from different means from publicly available data—the so-called big data or otherwise:

Sudden change or deviation from the usual flows of data in:

- International/domestic flights to-and-from certain cities
- Direction and intensity of traffic flow
- Increase of procurement of medical supplies
- Consumers' retail purchase patterns
- Movements or relocations of medical and emergency personnel
- Sharp growth of sentiments or certain topics from social media

Just like any disease, a macro-view of symptoms can be observed from people and their behaviours before a confirmed case emerged and officially reported to authority. There is always some time overhead or latency between the start of the first infection and mass infection. This observation period ensures the initial few infections are not of a singular or sporadic case in order to prevent unnecessary public panic if it were a false alarm. The length of the latency is complex, depending on the social–political structure of the city/national authority, usually from days to a week. While the authorities were waiting and monitoring the development of a potential outbreak from a small number, AI model that has been tapping on the vibe of the city beats round the clock, might have already sensed something unusual. For example, when a significant number of people started to show symptoms of an unknown disease, they would rant at the social media telling their circles of friends about their unwellness; those people and their friends and relatives would use search engines like Google, Bing and Baidu to seek information about the novel disease. This collective behaviour gives rise to surges of frequency of search keywords that could be picked up by web bots and Google Trend. Some web bots would be scrapping social blogs, tweets, opinions and comments posted on social media, harvesting hints of the illness-related sentiments and keywords, right from the patients and their peers.

Implementing this type of early warning prediction system requires a cooperative system of AI technologies. Its operation might have already been infiltrated into our daily lives without us knowing. The infiltration does not even intrude illegally into our privacy. Our modern society is accustomed to sharing and outreaching our private life in words, photos and videos, revealing our identities, background and even locations all the time. Similar to online advertising recommenders who collect logs of our online activities, these digital footprints are perfect ingredients to feed web bots, for them to understand trends and events of everybody's life. In the name of disease outbreak detection, the enabling AI technologies for hunting our information at the individual level include information retrieval [2], text mining [3] and NLP [4]. These three steps are conducted automatically running 24/7 across as many social media and news platforms as possible, for absorbing information relevant to a disease outbreak in high quantity and quality. The steps form an end to end process, taking the collected information spied online on each individual social media user, analysed and infer about a predicted hypothesis—a collective signal that an unknown disease is among the people, and they are getting increasingly concerned about it. To take a step for validating this hypothesis further, macro-view data analytics is applied, the so-called big data analytics [5] which massively collect big data feeds from CCTV, IoT, mobile phone usage data, GPS, voices, emails, ATM transactions and any form of digital communication and activities transferred online [6]. Similar AI algorithms but different in designs and scalability for functioning in big data infrastructure are used. The analytic results from both macro- and micro-levels are augmented, in order to predict an outcome with higher certainty. In addition to the three steps in the prediction process, popular data analytics with AI are anomaly detection and correlation analysis and often with visualization. Anomaly detection, sometimes known as outlier detection or deviation detection is a method of recognizing abnormal events which happened along a timeline of normal events. Often the detected abnormal events are suspicious and warrant investigation. The detected rare events may lead to grave consequences if they are ignored. Picking out the events which are characterized by extraordinary values can be done either simply by computing the interquartile range of the variables or clustering which groups similar data points together, for data that are of two-dimensional (variable of changing values over time) and multi-dimensional (many of those variables), respectively. The rare events will reveal themselves as outliers (data points that stay far from the median) with respect to the majority of data points, either in the form of box-plots or visual clusters. In anomaly detection, outliers will stand beyond a scale that is centred by an Interquartile Range (IQR). Firstly, all the data are used to compute IQR which is comprised of 25, 50 and 75% of all the data. Finding outliers from IQR is very common in descriptive statistics. It is a measure of statistical dispersion, being equal to the difference between the upper and lower quartiles. Some assumptions would have to be made by the users, to find outliers from the data: outliers are those data points that fall below $Q1$-*threshold* $\times$ IQR or above $Q3$ + *threshold* $\times$ IQR, where threshold typically takes a value of 1.5 which is called soft outlier threshold. It could be adjusted to be greater, called hard outlier threshold for identifying some very extreme outliers, e.g. at the value of 3 or larger (Fig. 3.1).

The IQR method is overly simple. The data points often are records of Tweets or sales patterns that would be well described by multiple attributes. In this case, clustering that makes use of Euclidean distance or Mahalanobis distance for measuring the non-linear similarity between data points is used. By the same concept as IQR, outliers are data points which fall outside of majority clusters. A visualization of outliers which lingering beyond the cluster that represents the main data distribution is shown in Fig. 3.2.

Correlation analysis is a statistical method which measures the closeness of the relationship between a pair of data series. It is useful for studying the relation between separate events which happen in pace at (almost) the same time or by (almost) the same trends. For predicting disease outbreak, often these two methods are used in

Fig. 3.1 Boxplot and a
probability density function
of a normal distribution of
$N(0, \sigma 2)$ population

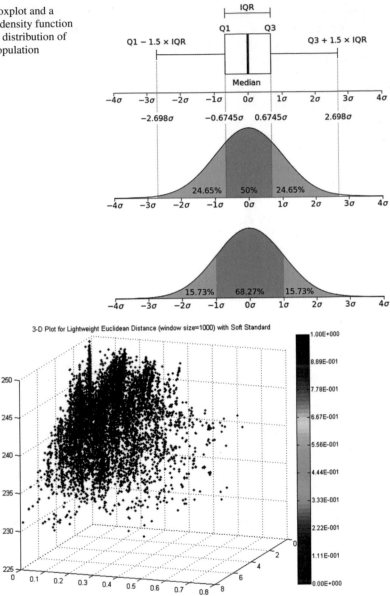

Fig. 3.2 Visualization of outliers detected by clustering using Euclidean Distance

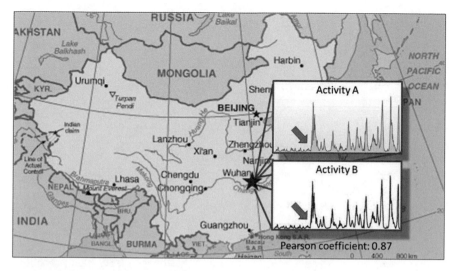

Fig. 3.3 Illustration of anomaly detection, correlation comparison and geo-map visualization

complementary to each other. For example, in a city it is detected that a surge of tweets complaining about their discomfort (or medical symptoms), at the same time people are panic-buying relevant symptoms-relief medicine from pharmacy stores. The rates of online posts and drug store purchases are correlated. Then it is pretty sure that some illness is going on in the population. These signals can be picked up by the prediction system and analysed using anomaly detection and correlation analysis. For decision support, the anomalies and their correlations could be visualized over a geographical map. An example is illustrated in Fig. 3.3 where two activities exhibited irregular patterns different from the past, and they arise at almost the same time same trends.

Being able to detect anomalies among the activities in a city triggers an alert. However, the prediction can be taken further from the moment and current situation to continuously predict about the future development of the outbreak. The latest ingredients from the data sources will continue to be tapped on, for further predicting how the outbreak will take place next, how many days before it will hit certain places, what the estimated number of infected cases will be and even how much damage it may cost. Further big data analytics could reference to the population of the nearby cities, the demographic details (percentage of vulnerable groups), the medical supports and intensity of social gatherings, hence the spreading rate, etc. These variables could be inputted to another prediction model which is formulated for extended prediction knowing that an outbreak is detected to be happening soon at a place. In this extended prediction process, there are a number of machine learning algorithms [7] that could be used, deep learning is one of the popular choices. This prediction process at the frontline requires the most up-to-date information which could come from the same data sources that were used to detect anomaly prior to the outbreak. Figure 3.4 shows a process diagram with two tiers of prediction modules.

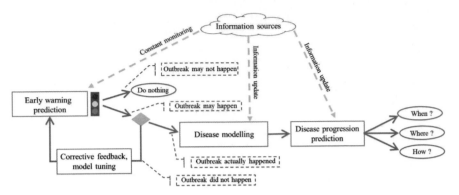

Fig. 3.4 A two-tier prediction model for predicting the next pandemic using big data

One is used for triggering an alert by continuous monitoring relevant activities. Once a potential outbreak is speculated to happen with a considerably high probability, the second prediction model will be launched to further analyse using the latest information available and predict a list of outcomes concerning the progress of the outbreak.

3.2   AI Predicts the Fate of COVID-19 Patients

Soon after the outbreak has begun, without exception, hospitals of every country are overwhelmed by many patients who are infected by the virus, causing huge stress on the medical teams. What if the likelihood of a COVID-19 patient developing into severe illness could be predicted? If the propensities of the clinical pathways for this novel disease could be predicted well, medical resources can be better allocated, managed and prepared in advance. Knowing the foreseen severe illness in advance means a more realistic estimation of demands in resources especially special equipment or those in tension which may require a long process for acquisition. The whole treatment process for every patient could be made more efficient.

Upon the urgency of needing an AI-supported clinical tool in predicting the fate of COVID-19 patients, a synergy is sparked between researchers from School of Medicine, New York University, USA and two Chinese hospitals, collaboratively develop a new AI prediction system [8]. During the project, they discovered that not all mild symptoms are equally important in turning a COVID-19 patient to severity of illness in a later stage. To most people's surprise, they observed that the popular symptoms such as high body temperature, early lung CT scans (before glass-like opacity is apparent), strength of body immunity and the patient's demographic details such as age, race, gender do not really predict well the consequence of serious disease. Testing out all possible variable factors, which are called predictors or attributes in data mining, over very limited number of patients at the beginning of the outbreak, they found that all the popular mild symptoms do not predict well. However, three somewhat surprising factors do link strongly to the development of severe illness in the later stage. They are surge in haemoglobin levels found in the body, muscle aching (myalgia) and the subtle fluctuation of presence of enzyme called alanine aminotransferase in the liver. When these three predictors are used together, a relatively good accuracy level at 80% can be achieved in predicting one of the later-stage illness known as Acute Respiratory Distress Syndrome (ARDS). In layman's term, ARDS is the difficulty of breathing which took many lives of COVID-19 patients at the end.

How this prediction can be done, which can attain up to 80% accuracy over a small available sample set using only three predictors? In AI, this is predictive analytics, which is about training up a representative model that recognizes the relations or mapping between the attributes of the dataset and the predicted outcome, which is simply binary—Yes, it will lead to ARDS or otherwise. The underlying relations at the predictive model could be highly non-linear considering that a number of attributes can take on very different values, out of many possible combinations, there is one that forms a strong decision path that points to the predicted outcome. The rest of the combinations and their links rather look random and meaningless (no strong link exists).

The predictive model would consist of two round of selections—feature selection as pre-processing step and random forest which selects the best performing decision tree from many other optional trees. Feature selection is basically a feature engineering process which transforms a full set of features with, however, maximum number of features (attributes) that describe the data to only a feature subset, that is, significant enough for making a reasonably accurate prediction. In the case of ARDS, the subset contains only three features, the liver enzyme, myalgia and haemoglobin level, that are sufficient to make an accurate prediction in lieu of the whole feature set which might contain other possible symptoms and patient's demographic details. It is known that given the number of maximum features is m, there is 2^m number of possible candidate feature subsets. For $m = 64$, the number of candidates is $2^{64} = 18446744073709551616$ (20 digits) which is an astronomical number. It implies that the search must cycle through that many times of repeating the tests over all the possible candidate subset by brute-force. An alternative search is by metaheuristic search or swarm search [9]. Several randomly chosen features are picked into a candidate subset at the beginning; using heuristics the candidate subset improves its selection of features in each round. The feature subset is refined in each round, until a predefined maximum number of iterations is reached or no more significant gain in the marginal improvement between successive cycles is observed. At each iteration, a slightly modified feature subset is put into the predictive model building process, for testing out the goodness of the current feature subset. The flowchart of swarm feature selection is shown in Fig. 3.5.

The iteration time varies according to the workflow depicted in Fig. 3.5. However, what most consuming probably is the core of the selection operation, namely, the 'classification model training' module. It basically builds a predictive model based on the input candidate feature subset each time. Each time after a predictive model is

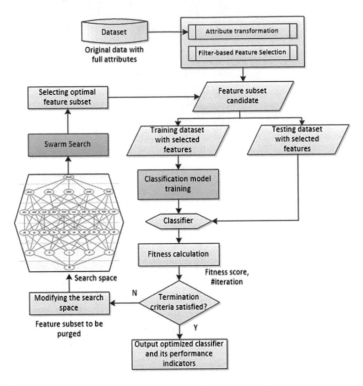

Fig. 3.5 Flowchart of swarm search-based feature selection method

built, it is put under test using the available testing data; the performance of the model is recorded as a fitness value which could be the average error in the prediction test using the candidate feature subset.Certain computing power requirement imposed on the hardware is required for fulfilling this iterative testing.

On the other hand, a Random Forest (RF) [10] which is an ensemble of decision trees in tournament is needed for assuring the highest possible level of accuracy in the final predictive model. RF is a competitive algorithm specialized in finding the best form of decision tree in doing classification task which tells apart the patients that will develop into ARDS from those otherwise. RF tries various combinations of model configuration parameters, different portions of training samples and even different features (which is unnecessary here since we have swarm search feature selection as pre-processing). It tries to exploit the memory space of the computer in trying out different individual decision trees which are dissimilar to each other, forming a collection of decision trees made up of different configurations. Then RF conducts a committee voting to vote for one that is more accurate than the rest of other individual trees, nominating that tree as a final winner. The winning tree is the best of all, taken as the final decision tree model at the end. In the context of using AI to predict ARDS consequence for COVID-19 patients, the final winning decision tree is used as decision support. Each branch of the final winning decision tree is traversed

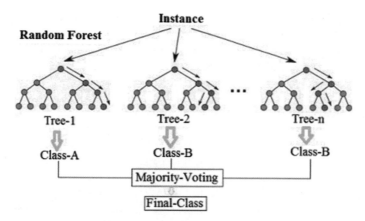

Fig. 3.6 Illustration of generating different optional trees in Random Forest

by testing each option at each tree nodes along the tree path, eventually after a series of chosen options, it leads to a conclusion at the leave (bottom level of the tree) indicating whether or not the patient will be suffering from ARDS. An illustration of RF is shown in Fig. 3.6 where each optional tree is built by using different portions of training samples, in order to generate a pool of different trees for performance selection. In this project, however, the training sample size is limited, instead different parameter values and configurations are tried, together with the swarm search feature selection, in finding out the best decision tree as the end output.

3.3   Finding the Most Accurate Predictive Analytics

Trends of disease spread can be monitored by data analytics and statistics. Predictive analytics which is a major branch of AI can forecast by regression and identify by classification where and how much healthcare demands are anticipated. So, resource planning, acquisition and allocation can be facilitated more precisely and timely. By knowing the spread patterns and fusing the trends with consideration of other social factors, intervention can be better applied. However, predictive analytics is not guaranteed to deliver perfect prediction every time, although it is known to do better than human educated guesses. Rarely a100% accuracy can always be achieved.

A tech giant Alibaba developed a one-stop AI system [11] solution at the urgency of relieving the overloads from the frontline healthcare workers. The AI system claims that an accuracy of 96% can be achieved in distinguishing between coronavirus infection in CT scans of patients from other pneumonia cases. The advantage of the AI system is more on the speed and efficiency which takes typically 20 s for a decision rather than a quarter of an hour when done by human experts which are heavily overloaded. The AI model is trained with 5000 empirical CT scans from confirmed coronavirus patients collected during the initial period of outbreak.

US military announced an AI algorithm [12], that is, able to predict infection 2 days ahead of clinical suspicion, before apparent symptoms can be confirmed, at accuracy level of 85%. The model is trained by using more forty thousand cases which are collected globally and 165 biomarkers. Early warning of a person who is likely to develop into COVID-19 patient, made possible by wearing wearable sensors that are strapped over the chest and wrists for biosignal monitoring. From the complex relations between the vital signal streams from each biomarker, the AI algorithm will know if the person will fall ill in the next 48 h before symptoms emerge. Again, in this technology, time is a priority for early warning and saving the potential risk of identifying a virus carrier that may infect other crew members if he is not detected early.

It can be seen that early prediction followed by detection, confirmation and intervention from Fig. 3.7 is essential to enhance the medical treatment process from one end to another. Predictive analytics plays an important role, despite speed and efficiency, accuracy is important. With the current glooming figures of over 2 millions infected cases and over 160 thousands deaths, even a slight percentage of errors from predictive analytics means putting thousands of lives at risk of false-negative detection. Section 3.2 discussed optimized feature selection and ensemble decision trees help sharpening the accuracy of a prediction model. However, these fine-tuning techniques are applicable to predictive analytics at individual level, i.e. predicting the outcome of a particular patient. The prediction is usually done by training–testing phases of repetition until a satisfactory level of accuracy could be reached; or else, the input variables, such as selection of training data, choice of method of feature selection, choice of predictive algorithm and its parameter values, should be re-tuned.

Timeline of COVID-19 disease progression		Predictive surveillance	Clinical surveillance
Infection	Hit by the virus, without even knowing	Early warning before symptoms appear	
Feeling unwell	Body starts to weaken		
Symptoms	Apparent symptoms arise, such as fever, body aching and dry cough	Prediction the likilihood of infection	
Home medication	Pain killer or symptom relief medicine (in the hope that mild symptoms may go away)	Oprional: Telemedicine remote consultation	
Hospital admission	Needing medical attendance		
Screening	Basic observation at triage, to determine the appropriate direction of treatment	Classify the patients into group (for decision support only)	Basic body check
Infection testing	Throat Swab Culture, Rapid Influenza Antigen, Blood Test, CT Scan, etc		Infection identified and confirmed
Treatment	Medication and other medical intervention, including respiratory aid and ICU if necessary	Predictive pathway (for decision support only)	Traditional clinicial pathways
Discharge	Leaving hospital because the patient is recovered or deceased	Accumulate medical history as record, for future predictive model improvement	

Time ↓

Fig. 3.7 Timeliness of AI predictive analytics in disease progression

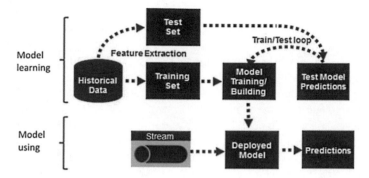

Fig. 3.8 The traditional training and testing process in building a predictive model from data feed for medical prediction

When a model is trained sufficiently to maturity, new data feed is subject to the model as unseen testing data to the model for making a prediction.

The train-and-test process shown in Fig. 3.8 is generic, suitable for predictive analytics for both individual patient and the trends of disease spread for a population. The advantage is the ability to observe the performance output at the end of the model training before it could be put into actual use. Knowing the performance and scoring them quantitively provides an opportunity for fine-tuning the prediction model. Being able to benchmark a prediction model is very important in this case, because we have several layers of uncertainty: not all algorithms generate good results; the model performance is sensitive to the training and testing data, sensitive to parameters and configuration of the model and features that characterize the data. Tuning up the best performing model is a tricky task because multiple health signals and variation in training records. This problem is worse especially in the beginning of the outbreak where the available samples are few and variation is high. But ironically a reliable model is more demanded for rushing out to the deployment at this crucial time.

The underlying reason for the difficulty in tuning up an accurate model is the fact that a set of heterogenous data are mixed and inputted as one training set to the model construction. These data come from logs of medical procedures, drugs and antibiotic administered, their responses from the body reaction, and the body conditions reflected from the vital signals. The interactions between these variables and their effects are complex, bound to be naturally non-linear in their relationship with respective to the predicted outcomes.

A methodology for finding the best AI algorithm is recently published, called Group of Optimized and Multi-source Selection (GROOMS) [13]. GROOMS is created with an objective of finding a model that gives the best prediction accuracy under the shortcoming of having limited available and little knowledge about the novel disease. GROOMS allows ensemble forecasting similar to random forest, by generating a group of forecasting models with parameter values tuned; some candidate models can take on several input data sources since medical forecasting often relies on multiple sources as mentioned above.

As shown in Fig. 3.9 GROOMS methodology allows loading in a small dataset sample which may be all that is available in the early time; passing them through three passages from top to bottom. A number of candidate models are tested on the data, each of which has its parameter values tuned to optimal. Some models are multiple regression which embrace multi-modal data from different sources. There are generally three types of forecasting algorithms in the AI family: 1) non-parametric models that have no parameter except a single input variable from a time-series input. 2) parametric models that have multiple parameters that are sensitive to performance and need to be tuned for the best performance. For instance, decision trees have parameters about splitting criteria and minimum or maximum number of nodes/depths of tree, etc. Neural networks have parameters about learning rate, momentum rate, network structure activation function, etc. 3) dual models—machine learning models that are sensitive to both of data input and the model parameters; they generally require most time and most difficult to tune.

The candidate models from the three passages are constructed, tuned, tested and performance is scored. This may repeat, however, times it takes, until each candidate model gets tuned up to its best performance. When they are ready, all the candidate models are subject to a committee voting assessment like a panel section. For regression style prediction models, the average fitting errors, e.g. RMSE is taken as a performance score. The panel selects a winner model which can produce a forecast

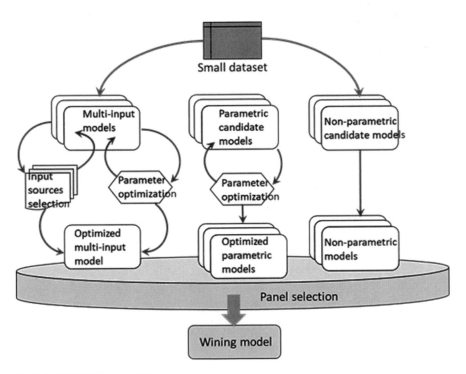

Fig. 3.9 GROOMS methodology

Fig. 3.10 GROOMS in action, evaluating AI algorithms in order from simple to complex

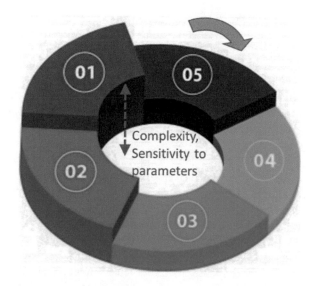

or prediction at the lowest error rate. The forecast or predicted outcome is therefore deemed to be one that is best available from what is available on hand.

How do data scientists go about using GROOMS given there are various sorts of machine learning and data analytics available in the big family of AI? The techniques differ in complexity, speed in modelling and sensitivity to parameter tuning, which can be roughly placed in five groups. The order of evaluating all the techniques is advocated as the sequence shown in Fig. 3.10. If time is not of constrained, all the techniques could be tried for selecting the best which may take days or weeks depending on the computing hardware available and the volume and dimension of the data. If time is urgent, especially during the critical moments of rescues when some scientific analysis is needed urgently, it is advised to progressively tested from simple techniques to sophisticated but time-consuming techniques.

The techniques are ranked in complexity in five groups, where Group 5 is the simplest, and Group 1 is the most complex. Although the exact time taken for each technique in each group is quite unpredictable, it is generally known that computation involves iteratively refinement and complex matrix operation would take much longer than basic statistical inference, e.g. moving average, which works over the data in just one pass. The five groups of techniques generally are as follows.

Group 05: Time-series forecasting by econometrics principles—this group of data analytics attempts to find a curve-fitting curve over the actual data curve, interpolating the fitted curve to the future horizon for estimating forecast. Popular choices are regression, auto-/exponential regression, integrative autoregression moving average, etc. Although this group is not the simplest among the five, they are fundamental and should attempted first as classical methods. The results are trustworthy in view of many statisticians.

Group 04: Basic data analytics—this group serves as a complementary role supporting the results of group 1 techniques and results. They expand the description of the data on the statistics landscape, by charting the statistics results. Common techniques are descriptive statistics, where the mean, median, min/max, variance and standard deviation are computed, frequency distribution, histograms, scatter-plots, box-plots, etc., e.g. average, min, max, the increments since yesterday or some days ago, rate of increases of suspected cases in comparison to cured cases, etc. These visualization charts, though basic, are some of the most popular techniques that most countries are using now to monitor and track the development of the virus spread. Government concern about the accelerating rate which is shown as the gradient of a curve of confirmed/suspected cases during the outbreak. The so-called flattening the curve means the gradient as daily increase is kept below certain threshold, so that the hospitals and medical infrastructure remain capable to treat new patients. It is alarming if ever the growth of the curve exceeds the threshold, implying that the medical system is collapsing no longer being able to handle new patients. The consequence is disastrous, as infected cannot be treated, they could only come home after refused by hospital, continue to infect their families and neighbours like a chain reaction. The threshold is a user-defined arbitrary variable that should be set according to the medical capacity of a country which is different country to country. The general rule of thumb is to keep the curve well under the threshold as much as possible imposing lockdown measure, discouraging and even forbidden anybody to travel out unnecessarily. Some of these typical charts are shown on COVID-19 dashboard, programmed in Tableau which is an interactive visualization software, in Fig. 3.11.

Group 03: Lightweight machine learning algorithms for forecasting—simple machine learning algorithms like those called 'lazy learners' or 'incremental learners' are used as base learners in forecasting. In contrast to conventional machine learning algorithms based on greedy-search, the incremental leaners learn to approximate the fitting curve to the actual curve, by updating the model on pass of data at a time. Incremental learners run fast on par with their counterparts, producing reasonably accuracy performance. Relatively they are also prone to misfitting by either overfitting or underfitting the training data. Tuning up the parameter properly is necessary for building a useful model.

Group 02: Complex machine learning algorithms for forecasting—complex machine learning algorithms are used as base-learner for doing forecasting. These algorithms in general are capable of recognizing and handling the non-linearity from complex data series that are twisted with jitters and large magnitudes of fluctuation. The model requires intensive parameter tuning too because the accuracy performance is very sensitive to the model configuration. For examples, SVM takes several important parameters each of which will impact greatly on the accuracy performance as well as the final outcome. Depending on the implementation of the algorithm, typical parameters are regularization variable of error term, kernel (poly, Sigmoid, rbf, or linear), degree of the kernel function for the polynomial (if the kernel = poly), gamma and initiation state, etc.

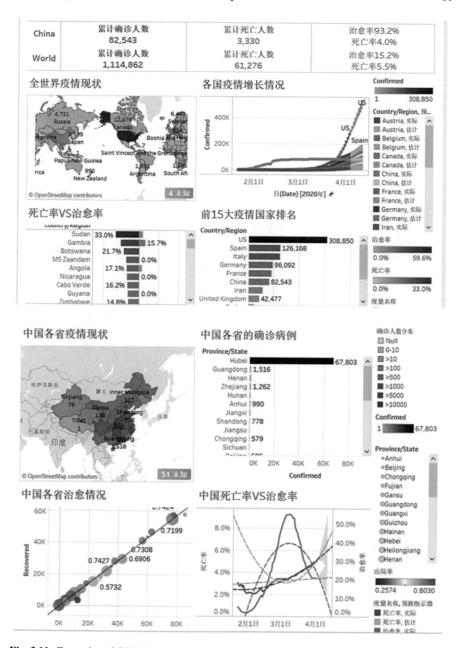

Fig. 3.11 Examples of COVID-19 dashboards using simple charts programmed in Tableau

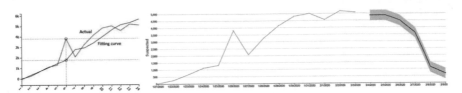

Fig. 3.12 Comparison of early forecasts by simple predictive analytics and the complex algorithm. Left: Holt-Winter, Right: Polynomial Neural Network

    Group 01: Complex machine learning algorithms with multiple regressions for forecasting—very non-linear machine learning model, such as neural network that takes many options of how the network structure can be configured and the associating parameters and activation function. Deep learning belongs to this category which has even more options in convolution feature maps set up in addition to the default neural network setup. This category is suitable for small and limited data but correlated data from multiple sources. For prediction of COVID-19 virus spread, forecasting in early stage is important; but data is scarce in short or very little history. Multiple regression may be used here, feeding in a collection of related data as inputs. Model tune-up involves the parameters for the model itself and the pre-processing of a group of time-series.

    Figure 3.12 shows a comparative forecasting example over the early time-series of daily increase of confirmed COVID-19 cases. The forecasts are made by Holt-Winter algorithm which is a popular econometric from Group 5 and Polynomial Neural Network with multiple regression from Group 1. It can be seen that the forecasts by the two groups of methods lead to totally different outcomes. The Holt-Winter method from Group 1 placed too much empathizes on the trend of the data curve, the forecast is almost a straight line that follows the same gradient from the past records. In contrast, the Polynomial Neural Network from Group 5 that inputs the other relevant data series offers a reasonable forecast curve with a gradual downward trend and few small turns. At the end of writing, it is known that the daily increase cases for China have dropped to a single-digit figure close to none. The Group 5 algorithm predicted so several weeks ago prior to the actual drop that really had happened. In summary, one must be careful in choosing the right AI algorithm in prediction especially if the prediction involves life and death. If it is urgent, lightweight approaches could be used. If time is allowed, it worth investing the time spent on tuning up the parameters as well as considering other relevant data series together, for a quality forecasting model,

3.4 Predicting the Virus Spread by SIR and SEIR Models

In epidemiology, mathematical modelling is used to estimate the spread of the disease considering important and dynamic variables which are inter-depending on one another. Unlike time-series forecasting which is purely based on historical records from which a forecast is projected to the future horizon, mathematical modelling based on compartment model is used involving three or more inter-link factors. The accuracy of prediction from time-series forecasting assumes the future situations remain unchanged, which is unrealistic. The forecast is merely a projection of what happened in the past, following up the same trend from the fitted curve which is again inferred based on history.

The mathematical modelling that is favoured by epidemiologists is inherited from the concept of compartment model. Compartment model has been used to simulate transport of quantified items from one state to another, often within a closed-loop and bounded space. For example, moving one kilogram of ice from a freezer room to a kitchen at room temperature, you will have 1 kg of less ice from the freezer room but increase by 1.091 litre of water, assuming it is a closed system without evaporation, leaks or vents through which the material will escape to elsewhere. A simulation can be set up thereby the room temperature in kitchen could be tested as a variable against the amount of water as liquid that exists in the kitchen compartment. By the same analogy, a simulation can be set up to study the inter-relationships between the three major variables of which their existences are interlinking and proportional. The three common variables in epidemiology are Susceptibles (S)—how many people are healthy but susceptible to virus infection, Infected (I)—how many people who were healthy and now become infected and Recovered (R)—how many people who were infected now have recovered. They are equivalent within a confined system. It is noted that the transitions between these three variables are unidirectional (S → I → R) and the relations are proportional. The more people are infected the less healthy ones we got, infested and recovered numbers are somewhat correlated. Taking time as a system variable, as days pass by, one can observe how many people remain susceptible, infested and recovered. At any point of time, the values of the three variables can be projected and observable along the horizon of future days. For example, given a fixed population, we will know the numbers for S, I and R, and their interaction as time progresses, when we define some changing rates from S to I and I to R. The rates are known as contagious rate (or reproduction rate) and recovering rate, respectively.

The S.I.R. model was theorized as a mathematical model by Kermack and McKendrick in 1927 [14], coined after the definitions of the three compartments S, I and R. SIR model is one of the most fundamental models, based on which other variants are developed to model epidemics and pandemics of different characteristics [15]. Taking time t (in days) as a natural and discrete variable which will pass day after day regardless of whatever will happen on earth, the dependent variables in the model are defined as a function of time:

- $S(t)$ = number of susceptible persons at time t. Everybody is assumed to be born susceptible to virus infection. For COVID-19, it is assumed that susceptible (healthy) individuals who were infected and once they managed to recover, will be immuned. So everybody can only be infected once in their lifetime in this scenario although there are some rare cases as exception that a same person gets infested twice or more.

- $I(t)$ = number of infected persons at time t. These are the people who had contracted the disease and able to pass on the disease to susceptible people, regardless of symptomatic or asymptomatic. Once infected, the individual will only move on to the R stage, as a matter of time. I_0 is the zero patient, $I(0)$ is originally how many of such zero patient exists at the beginning. Usually $I(0)$ is unknown or by default set to 1.
- $R(t)$ = the number of recovered persons at time t. R patients are those came from I but either recovered or died at the end. In either way, R patients will not be infected again, neither can they become S nor I anymore.

As such, converting the functions in number above to percentage, we have $s(t) = \frac{S(t)}{N}$, $i(t) = \frac{I(t)}{N}$, and $r(t) = \frac{R(t)}{N}$, where N is the number of population which remains unchanged throughout the simulation. Births and migration within the simulation period are not considered in the model. Then summing up the percentages $s(t) + i(t) + r(t) = 1$ in the close-loop system, where $s(t)$ and $i(t)$ are directly inverse proportional to each other, $i(t)$ and $r(t)$ are associated with a decay function. The model requires additional assumptions to maintain the validity. $S(t)$ will only decrease or remain the same number since an outbreak started, the rate of decline is subject to the number of susceptibles who can remain isolated, the number infested who can infest, and the intensity of contact level between the remaining susceptibles and the increasing number of infested. Let β be the number of contacts through which each infected person will infect susceptibles per day, assuming that the virus is absolutely contagious. That means once any single disease carrier contacted the previously unexposed susceptible, he will be infected for sure. β is known as a reproduction rate by which the disease spreads. At the beginning, everybody is susceptible to COVID-19 (assuming nobody is born immune). If β is equal to 1, each infested will pass the disease on to a susceptible. If β is smaller than 1, the outbreak will not sustain because the number of people to be infected will be less than the number of existing infested in the future; the pandemic will die out sooner or later. But if β is greater than 1, the population will experience an exponential growth of infection.

By referring to past experiences of similar respiratory pandemics, the reproduction rate β for COVID-19 is estimated to be around 1.5 and in the worst scenario β can be up to 4. It was conservatively calibrated to 2 in the initial two months of outbreak since mid-December 2019. By $\beta = 2$, the initial infested person would spread the disease to two others, each of these two others will continue to spread to another two others, and so forth the disease propagates. The growth rate of the disease spread is drastically as sharp as exponential, but it is not uncommon in the early stage of outbreak. However, assume no control is applied to stop or slow down the spread, more than a thousand people could be infected starting from only one person after 10 days. Given another 10 days down the road, the total number of infected people be over a million. And this will continue to multiply to tens or hundreds of millions in a worst-case scenario in the near future. Such sharp rises can be seen in some countries in terms of death tolls in Fig. 3.13. The death tolls are very much proportional to the

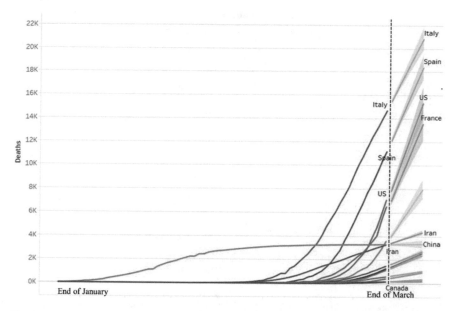

Fig. 3.13 Sharp rises of death tolls in US and European countries at the beginning of COVID-19 (data source: https://www.tableau.com/covid-19-coronavirus-data-resources)

number of infected patients. It is known about 5% in average in the world; however, this varies from country to country. Figure 3.14 shows a tornado chart of the top highest Case Fatality Rate (CFR) as of end of March 2020. Although there are many factors that lead to death, such as age, strength of body immunity and pre-existing illness conditions, the increase of number of infected people has a direct impact on the capacity of hospital upon which the chances of a patient's recovery or otherwise rely on. To the end of this, keeping the number of infected patients under control while protecting the susceptibles is a prime objective, and S.I.R model is going to inform us about the future scenarios of how far we are from these two equivalent targets.

To simulate the dynamic of the S.I.R. model, we let the transition probability from compartments S to I as $\frac{\beta}{N} \times \omega$ where ω is infective index (having $\omega = 1$ means for certain each contact will get a susceptible infected), and from compartments I to R, the transition probability is governed by γ which is mortality rate or removal rate. γ is the average number of infected patients who recovered or died per day over the total number of people who are currently infected on the same day. The dynamics of the S.I.R. system mainly depend on two forces—how contagious that a susceptible became infected and how soon an infected individual can be removed from the system. The removal rate is directly hinged on how much capacity a medical system can provide in quickly testing, identifying and confirming the suspected individual, and perhaps quarantine them in time before he goes around and infects other people. This issue relates to the availability of test-kits and the efficiency of the

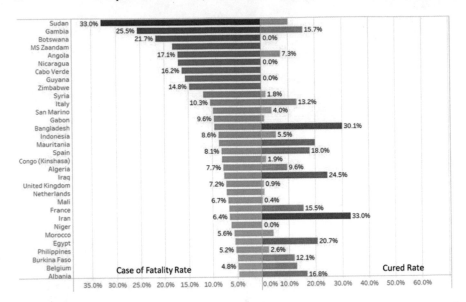

Fig. 3.14 Top-ranked countries with highest CFR in COVID-19 pandemic (*Data source* https://www.tableau.com/covid-19-coronavirus-data-resources)

medical team, as well as the demands for these resources depending on the number of infected people. In the previous chapters, AI and technologies have been discussed in improving the medical capacity and efficiency. Nevertheless, the medical capacity assuming is a precious resource which shall not be overloaded even we have the best AI and best medical team. Keeping β as low as possible is imperative here. On average, $\beta \times s(t)$ number of new infected people are generated every day. These newly increasing infested people who supposedly need medical attention and the additional supply of medical resources are sitting on a seesaw; unfortunately, medical resources cannot be easily increased in a short time, but the newly infected people pile up in thousands every day in some countries. To make matter worse, infected patients who are rejected from hospitals due to over-capacity may roam around or at home infecting family members or other caregivers.

The S.I.R. model is constituted by the kinetic energies of three equations—the Susceptible equation, the Recovered equation and the Infected Equation in Eqs. (3.1), (3.2) and (3.3) as below:

$$\frac{ds}{dt} = -\beta \times s(t) \times i(t) \tag{3.1}$$

$$\frac{dr}{dt} = \gamma \times i(t) \tag{3.2}$$

$$\frac{di}{dt} = \beta \times s(t) \times i(t) - \gamma \times i(t) \tag{3.3}$$

$$\frac{ds}{dt} + \frac{di}{dt} + \frac{dr}{dt} = 0 \tag{3.4}$$

Equation (3.4) shows that the S.I.R. would have to remain balanced as an equivalent closed-loop system. So, for an example of setting up a S.I.R. model for COVID-19 outbreak that started on the first day in Wuhan, the city has a population of 11.08 million; assume there were 10 people who were infected and nobody had died of or recovered from the disease yet on the first day of outbreak. $S(0) = 11,080,000$; $I(0) = 0$; $R(0) = 0$. The complete S.I.R. model would therefore be

$$\begin{aligned}
\frac{ds}{dt} &= -\beta \times s(t) \times i(t) &\leftarrow& \qquad s(0) = 1 \\
\frac{di}{dt} &= \beta \times s(t) \times i(t) - \gamma \times i(t) &\leftarrow& \quad i(0) = 9.03 \times 10^{-7} \\
\frac{dr}{dt} &= \gamma \times i(t) &\leftarrow& \qquad r(0) = 0
\end{aligned} \tag{3.5}$$

In the early days of the outbreak, the coronavirus was novel. It is an educated guess initially to assume the values for the parameters β and γ to start the model. Then as the spread progresses and more information is collected, the values for these two variables would be adjusted to fit the actual scenarios. For an example and sake of illustration of how S.I.R. model works, the following assumptions are made: a small city with population of 100,000; an infected patient has an average timespan of 25 days of being infectious until either he recovered or passed away, so $\gamma = 0.04$; everyday every infested carrier will infest between 2 and 5 susceptible people; therefore, a varying β is adjustable in the S.I.R. model such that $\beta = 1, 2, 3, 4$ and 5. Figure 3.15 shows four possible outcomes generated by the S.I.R. model when β varies from 1 to 5.

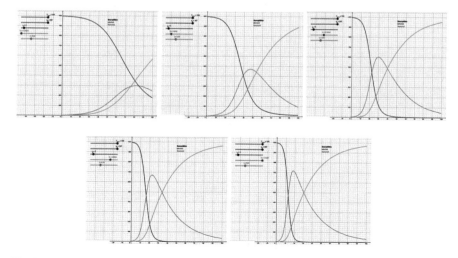

Fig. 3.15 Predicted scenarios by S.I.R. model with varying $\beta = 1, 2, 3, 4$ and 5 per population per day

It is noted that the output of the S.I.R. has three curves representing the future forecasts of the number of susceptibles, infested and recovered, respectively, on the horizon of future days. Mainly, these three curves depict the developments of the virus outbreak in different level of human contacts by β, starting with a small number of infested people escalates to a large number in a length of time. The red curves which represent the number of infested people are rising at a high rate, the more number of contacts per carrier per day, the sharper the gradient of the trajectory is. In all the four cases of simulation results, the trajectories will peak at different heights but sooner or later the curves slope down gradually due to the running out of fresh susceptibles to be infected and the recovery of those that were infected earlier. It is obvious that when the contact level of the population is set to minimum, the area under the susceptibles curve remains large. That is, the situation that every government wants to achieve, by keep most of the population spare from being infected. The other important point to be observed from the S.I.R. output is that the bell curves of the infected which may not be perfectly symmetrical should be kept as flat as possible. Or else it will exceed certain threshold where the hospital capacity is at maximum, once the curve goes beyond the threshold the hospital starts to get overloaded. If this situation is not remedied, the medical infrastructure will collapse and the frontline nurses and doctors in hospital get infected too as protective supplies run out and overworked to fatigue.

At all costs, the S.I.R. is telling us it is extremely mandatory to keep β at bay, preferably down to zero if possible though it means massive shut down in towns and cities, economy will be damaged. Assuming new vaccine will not be available any time in near future, social lockdown by social distancing, which is proven to be an effective measure, is necessary to keep a majority of population safe and wait for the virus to die out. Therefore, an important component in the S.I.R. model is missing, and the model needs to be extended to accommodate a compartment for the incubation period as 14 days is typical for COVID-19 and social distancing. Social distancing not only helps to keep β low by cutting down non-essential human interaction, but it also provides a space and time buffer for the person who was infected to seek medical help before he becomes infectious by his symptoms such as coughing. When social distancing is enforced, the just infested person as soon as he feels unwell, he would call CDC or any COVID-19 hotline. Thereafter, medical team would arrive his house, test him and escort him to hospital for quarantine during his home-safe period under national lockdown. This would result in early treatment and higher chance of successful cure. Furthermore, this latency provides opportunity for AI to help, such as telemedicine, timely detection as suspected cases and optimized hospital resource preparation.

To embrace this incubation or onset period of COVID-19 infection, S.I.R. model is, hence, modified to S.E.I.R model [16] which is suitable for inclusion of a latency period for COVID-19 between the compartments of Susceptible to Infected. Mathematically, for S.E.I.R. model, let $E(t)$ be the number of people per day exposed to the virus, infected but not infectious yet. $e(t)$ is the corresponding ratio of $E(t)$ per day per population. The mean latent period and the mean infectious period for COVID-19 are assumed to be $\frac{1}{\alpha}$ and $\frac{1}{\gamma}$ respectively, β is a rate that changes in time as

$\beta(t)$ where β_0 is the initial β value, and μ is the birth and death rates which are equal. The same assumption which states that no vaccine is available, and the recovered patients are permanently immune apply here. The additional Exposed equation and the other modified equations are defined as follow:

$$\frac{ds}{dt} = \mu - \beta(t) \times s(t) - \mu \times s(t) \tag{3.6}$$

$$\frac{de}{dt} = \beta(t) \times s(t) \times i(t) - (\mu + \alpha) \times e(t) \tag{3.7}$$

$$\frac{di}{dt} = \alpha \times e(t) - (\mu + \gamma) \times i(t) \tag{3.8}$$

$$\frac{ds}{dt} + \frac{de}{dt} + \frac{di}{dt} + \frac{dr}{dt} = 0 \tag{3.9}$$

$$\frac{\alpha \times \beta_0}{(\mu + \gamma)(\mu + \alpha)} = R_0 \tag{3.10}$$

R_0 is a significant indicator informing us how contagious the virus is [17]. It is known as Reproduction rate in S.E.I.R. model, defined by the mean number of susceptibles that an infected person will spread the virus to per day. So far, the exact reproduction rate for COVID-19 is not known yet, but it is estimated from the existing data from WHO to be ranging from 2 to 2.6. The rate differs from country to country which depends also on the preventative strategy applied by the government of that country. Comparing to COVID-19, the reproduction rate for seasonal flu is just about 1 that means an infected person will continue to infect another 1 or 2 persons only. SARS has reproduction rate at 3 which is more contagious and more deadly than COVID-19. SARS is very contagious only from the second week onwards after the symptoms appeared. In contrast, COVID-19 patient who first contracted the decease will become contagious immediately, symptoms then will appear 1 or 2 days later. Between the time prior to 48 hours, he got the symptoms and went to the hospital to be tested, he could potentially infect anybody that he will be in contact with. By using the S.E.I.R. model, it shows that this latency period is dangerous and R_0 can be subsided significantly by social distancing. The following screen-captures show the progression of COVID-19 spread, in the cases of 0 isolation, 80% isolation and 100% isolation, in Fig. 3.16. Mainly it shows how important isolation is. The simulation is programmed and hosted on a website, with URL: https://www.trackc orona.live/isolation. The simulation shows how sclf-isolation, enforced quarantine for suspected patients and social distancing contribute to 'flattening the curve' of COVID-19 pandemic.

In the near future, it is anticipated that the modelling of virus pandemic behaviours would be aided by AI for more precise estimating the ideal lockdown period. It is known that too short the period, the pandemic may re-bounce, too long the lockdown will harm deeper the economy driving high the unemployment rate and recession,

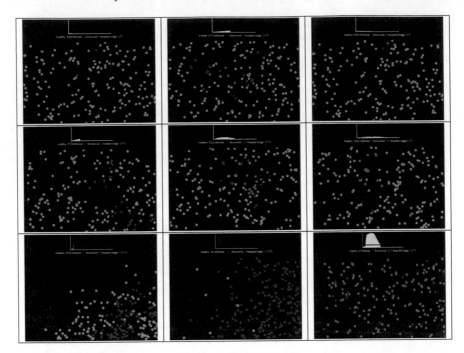

Fig. 3.16 Simulation of COVID-19 pandemic progress by S.E.I.R. model with (top) 100% social distancing, (middle) 80% social distancing, (below) no social distancing

etc. It could be formulated as a multi-objective optimization model by AI, in such a way that the death toll, the infected rate, the economy damage, the lockdown period and the necessary resources to fight the virus be minimized, but the number of susceptibles be maximized, saving life at the lowest costs, choosing intelligently the right mix of preventative strategies.

AI can also play a significant role in predicting more accurately the outcomes than simple mathematics models, being able to simulate the behaviours of the pandemic with more details using supercomputers. A recent work on decision support by stochastic simulation for resource allocation to fight COVID-19 is published [18]. Large-scale simulation by AI and superior computing hardware could be conducted along this direction. Moreover, AI has been used for drug discovery, drug design and drug testing which helps speeding up the R&D of COVID-19 vaccine [19].

References

1. Bowles J (2020) How Canadian AI start-up BlueDot spotted Coronavirus before anyone else had a clue, Diginomica, March 10, 2020, Accessed 18 April 2020
2. Nagypál G (2005) Improving information retrieval effectiveness by using domain knowledge stored in ontologies. In: Meersman R, Tari Z, Herrero P (eds) On the Move to Meaningful

Internet Systems 2005: OTM 2005 Workshops. OTM 2005. Lecture Notes in Computer Science, vol 3762. Springer, Berlin, Heidelber

3. Mohd Sharef N, Kasmiran KA (2012) Examining text categorization methods for incidents analysis. In: Chau M, Wang GA, Yue WT, Chen H (eds) Intelligence and security informatics. PAISI 2012. Lecture Notes in Computer Science, vol 7299. Springer, Berlin, Heidelberg

4. Tosey P, Mathison J (2009) What is NLP? The 'Six Faces' of the field. In: Neuro-linguistic programming. Palgrave Macmillan, London

5. Mohammed M, Hissam A, Mohammed T, Anya SO, Applications of big data analytics: trends, issues, and challenges, Springer, 2018. ISBN: 978-3-319-76471-9

6. Tromblay DE, Spying: Assessing US Domestic Intelligence Since 9/11, Lynne Rienner Publishers, February 25, 2019, ISBN: 978-1626377806

7. Alessa A, Faezipour M (2018) A review of influenza detection and prediction through social networking sites. Theor Biol Med Model 15:2. https://doi.org/10.1186/s12976-017-0074-5

8. Jiang X, Coffee M, Bari A, Wang J, Jiang X et al (2020) Towards an artificial intelligence framework for data-driven prediction of coronavirus clinical severity. CMC-Comput Mater Continua 63(1):537–551

9. Fong S, Deb S, Yang X, Li J (2014) Feature selection in life science classification: Metaheuristic Swarm search. IT Professional 16(4), 24–29

10. Bhadra P, Yan J, Li J et al (2018) AmPEP: Sequence-based prediction of antimicrobial peptides using distribution patterns of amino acid properties and random forest. Sci Rep 8:1697. https://doi.org/10.1038/s41598-018-19752-w

11. Greene T (2020) Alibaba's new AI system can detect coronavirus in seconds with 96% accuracy, TNW, 2 March 2020. Accessed 19 April 2020

12. Boyd A (2019) Military Algorithm Can Predict Illness 48 Hours Before Symptoms Show, Next Government, 24 Oct 2019. Accessed 19 April 2020

13. Fong SJ, Li G, Dey N (2020) Rubén González Crespo, Enrique Herrera-Viedma, Finding an accurate early forecasting model from small dataset: a case of 2019-nCoV novel coronavirus outbreak. IJIMAI 6(1):132–140

14. Kermack WO, McKendrick AG (1927) A contribution to the mathematical theory of epidemics. proceedings of the royal society a: mathematica., Phys Eng Sci 115 (772): 700. Bibcode:1927RSPSA.115..700 K. https://doi.org/10.1098/rspa.1927.0118.JSTOR94815

15. Vynnycky, Emilia; White, Richard G. An Introduction to Infectious Disease Modelling. Retrieved 2016–02-15. An introductory book on infectious disease modelling and its applications

16. Aron JL, Schwartz IB (1984) Seasonality and period-doubling bifurcations in an epidemic model. J Theor Biol 110:665–679

17. Sanche S, Lin YT, Xu C, Romero-Severson E, Hengartner N, Ke R (2020) High contagiousness and rapid spread of severe acute respiratory syndrome Coronavirus 2, EID Journal 26(7), 2020, ISSN: 1080-6059

18. Fong SJ, Li G, Dey N, Crespo RG, Herrera-Viedma E (2020): Composite monte carlo decision making under high uncertainty of novel coronavirus epidemic using hybridized deep learning and fuzzy rule induction. Appl Soft Comput 9:106282

19. Le TT, Andreadakis Z, Kumar A, Román RG, Tollefsen S, Saville M, Mayhew S (2020, The COVID-19 vaccine development landscape, Nature Reviews Drug Discovery, 9 April 2020, ISSN 1474-1784

Chapter 4
Conclusion

This book shows a buffet of artificial intelligence applications from drone to deep learning and from data analysis to the prediction of next pandemic disease along with its drug discovery. Today the entire globe is under the threat of COVID-19 affecting around 200 countries. The death toll reported in these highly affected countries has become catastrophic. Countries next in line where the pandemic is still in the second stage is closely monitored so as to check and create a barrier where there lies a severe chance of community spread. Here, close monitoring of sensitive regions using drones and modelling of the prediction mechanism to visualize the extent and severity of the spread of the disease within the community is highly required. Effective usage of drones has been reported encompassing community monitoring during lockdown to sanitization of the highly susceptible and the next probable hotspots. On the other hand, data analysis plays a pivotal role to understand the nature and the potential ability of community spreading. Although several drugs, which are administered to treat some major diseases in the developing nations are currently undergoing clinical trials and various tests for their response towards COVID-19. Although several promising results have come to the fore, nailing down to the vaccine is still an up-hill task.

Prediction of the risk of infection, its severity and nature of spread is attained by implementing machine learning models based on risk factors such as age, pre-existing disease, general habit and hygiene, frequency of social interactions, climate and socio-economic structures. The application of wearable body sensing devices also has a major impact in providing significant alerts by closely monitoring underlying health conditions. The self-triage system, m-health applications and AI assisted chatbots also play significant roles to help anxious patients. However, the reliability of several chatbots, m-health apps, etc. has been found to be highly questionable being linked to untrustworthy third-party sources with major privacy issues.

Artificial Intelligence is marching towards maturity. However, the masses are yet to acknowledge and adapt the advanced technologies developed by the medical researches. The pandemic like COVID-19 actually serves as a catalyst to develop the algorithm for modern viral disease detection mechanism and life-saving drug discovery. Several government-aided and private research institutes and funding agencies are coming forward to patronize research on drug discovery, severity measurement, PPE suit development, mask and sanitizer production, etc. Several prototypes and concepts have been tested, data collected and analysed. All the valuable information has been put to real-life test through this pandemic. The positive responses received from nations, which implemented AI techniques to curb and control the disease, indicate that this concept has paved the path towards restricting the spread of the pandemic along with suggesting standardized techniques for detection and monitoring of life-threatening diseases. Although this has been a panic-stricken journey, lots of valuable experience has been learned and practiced.

Anticipating a future where AI applications will evolve and enhance to serve the mankind.

Printed in the United States
By Bookmasters